# TORN
# ILLUSIONS

*ONE WOMAN'S
TRAGIC EXPERIENCE
WITH THE
SILICONE CONSPIRACY*

# TORN ILLUSIONS

*ONE WOMAN'S TRAGIC EXPERIENCE WITH THE SILICONE CONSPIRACY*

**Pamela Stott-Kendall**

**NEW HORIZON PRESS**
**Far Hills, New Jersey**

Requests for permission should be addressed to:
New Horizon Press
P.O. Box 669
Far Hills, NJ 07931

Stott-Kendall, Pamela.
        Torn Illusions : One woman's tragic experience with the silicone conspiracy

Library of Congress Catalog Card Number: 93-61692

ISBN: 0-88282-090-7 (hc)
ISBN: 0-88282-097-4 (pb)
New Horizon Press

Manufactured in the U.S.A.

1998 1997 1996 1995 1994 / 5 4 3 2 1

# AUTHOR'S NOTE

These are the actual experiences and history of Pamela Stott-Kendall, and this book reflects her opinion of the past, present and future. The personalities, events, actions and conversations portrayed within the story have been reconstructed from her memory, extensive interviews and research, utilizing court documents, letters, personal papers, press accounts and the memories of participants. In an effort to safeguard the privacy of certain individuals, the author has changed their names and, in some cases, altered otherwise identifying characteristics. Events involving the characters happened as described; only minor details have been altered.

# ACKNOWLEDGMENTS

Many have participated in making possible this publication, and I am greatly indebted to all, but several are especially due a heartfelt thank you.

Without Dr. Ira Finegold's unflagging support and assistance, his knowledgeable medical contributions, as well as his faith in my ability to carry out the task, this book may not have become a reality.

A few close friends have also played an important part in the outcome of my story. Importantly, Teresa St. Forte's care during the early days of silicone illness, enabled my survival during my incapacitation. Wendy Markwell Mallock is another whose friendship throughout the years actually resulted in an introduction to my future publishing agent, Mr. Bernard Kurman of Rights Unlimited, New York. As my agent, he was instrumental in the achievement of my goal. His trust that I could indeed write, and then publish my experiences and research, remained unswerving and provided me with the encouragement necessary in order to complete the project.

# TORN ILLUSIONS

Nancy Hartoin, a professor and writer from Winter Park, Florida, aided my struggle to recover my health and gave me courage in reaching this ultimate destination.

Sharon Goldstein, a college professor of English, has encouraged me to stay on course and offered much editorial advice. Also, Carrie Gulbrandsen and Richard Cherskov contributed a great deal of effort.

Included in my thank you are the countless medical professionals whose research comprised the basis for this publication. In particular, I wish to thank Dr. Pierre Blias of Ottawa, Canada. His immense knowledge concerning silicone implants proved invaluable, and I sincerely appreciate Dr. Blais' generosity when answering the many questions that I frequently asked. Dr. Don Roach of Miami, Florida, was also generous with both his time and his research.

To my publisher Joan Dunphy and her staff at New Horizon Press, I extend my praise for the help received along with an equal and ample amount of gratitude. Only with Joan's support was the publication of this book realized, and I am truly indebted. A special thank you goes to John Chambers, former senior editor of McGraw-Hill. John's interest in the silicone story benefited the final stages of editing.

In closing, not to be forgotten are the thousands of anonymous women whose suffering necessitated the writing of our story, your spirit is included within *Torn Illusions*.

# CONTENTS

# INTRODUCTION

*by*
*Ira Finegold, M.D.*

The book you are about to read details the quest of a courageous woman who sought to discover the nature of her illness despite the many physicians who felt this illness did not exist. Not only does Pamela Kendall take you through her own sad, mysterious illness and its eventual diagnosis and treatment, but she also expands her personal journey to reveal the devastating effects of silicone-gel implants on other women. She details how the scientific data related to silicone breast implants have been kept hidden from both the consumer and the physician.

Her illness has exacted a heavy toll on her life. This includes the dissolution of her marriage, the loss of her job, virtually years of being an invalid, multiple hospitalizations and many hours spent with physicians seeking an answer to her illness. She has also gained a great deal from this experience and has been triumphant in waging a war to find out what made her ill and how she could restore her health. This effort has strengthened her resolve, and, at this point, her health is so much improved that she has written this book in order to tell her story to the many women who still are ill and do not know where to seek help.

She also acts as a source of information and compassion as part of a network of women who have suffered from silicone-associated disease (SAD). Thus, she has become a much needed "angel of mercy," if you will, in helping women sort out this illusive illness.

It all began with a so-called mysterious illness and a puzzling chemical odor. I first saw Mrs. Kendall when she was referred to me by another physician, Dr. Jay Sanders, a well-known, astute clinician. At that time, he was involved with administrative medicine and was no longer seeing private patients. He referred her to me for continuing care and evaluation.

I am a board-certified allergist/immunologist with a background in research. While in medical school, I became interested in immunology through my research at the pathology department of the University of Chicago School of Medicine (now the Pritzer School of Medicine). There, I conducted research on the growth of tumors in mice. This led to published reports on how to interfere with host's (mouse) resistance and make the tumor grow larger by immunologic means.

As part of this research program, I received a Masters Degree in pathology as well as my medical degree with honors. I began internal medicine residency and, after two years, became an associate at the Cancer Institute of the Immunology Branch of the National Institute of Health (NIH). There, I continued immunologic research showing that certain cells in an artificial laboratory experiment can produce immunoglobulins. It was there that Dr. Sanders and I were part of the same team and co-authored a research paper.

I subsequently published other research findings on the presence of immunoglobulins from cells derived from an African tumor called Burkitt's Lymphoma. At that point, we knew that this was related to the Epstein Barr virus disease, and, in fact, some of the cells that I worked with had originally been established as continuous cell cultures by Epstein.

While at NIH, I decided to combine my immunology background with my internal medicine training, so I selected to enter

# TORN ILLUSIONS

the field of allergy/immunology. After receiving an additional fellowship in allergy and immunology, I began private practice of that specialty. While most of the diseases I encountered were asthma, hay fever, hives and so forth, every so often patients would present me with unusual illnesses for diagnosis. Thus, while Mrs. Kendall did not come in with "hay fever," she came in with an illness somewhat different and much more devastating.

I view the allergist/immunologist as a detective. The job of an allergist is to hear the detailed history, then, combined with a physical examination and diagnostic tests, seek to fit the data to a particular disease. Allergists/immunologists are unique in that, in order to be Board Certified in their field, they must first be certified in internal medicine and pediatrics.

Mrs. Kendall came to me with bizarre and unusual symptoms. Initially, I took the point of view that, based on her symptoms, I would try to rule out any known illness that fit the pattern of her problems. We explored metabolic, endocrinologic and neurologic possibilities with no conclusive results.

Early on, when she told me about her silicone implants, I had a suspicion that these were foreign bodies that could cause immune reactions. From my previous work in immunology, I had a great deal of respect for how the human body treats foreign substances and to what lengths it will go to purge itself of what does not belong. Sometimes this purging or reaction process, where the body attempts to get rid of the invader (whether this be a virus that infects the body and then continues to grow within the body or a foreign substance such as an implant or a transplant), is actually worse than the disease or problem caused by the foreign invader.

In the beginning, I was somewhat skeptical that all of Mrs. Kendall's symptoms were caused by the silicone implants, but I kept running into diagnostic dead ends when I sought other causes for her complaints. I recall telephoning her plastic surgeon while she was in the hospital incapacitated. I told him that I wasn't sure what caused her illness, but that I knew she would never be well unless we took out the implants.

# TORN ILLUSIONS

The subsequent course of events is detailed in this book. However, as I have said before, now that Mrs. Kendall is free of her implants, she continues to progress in her recovery. Not only is the case for her illness being caused by silicone-associated disease (SAD) based on her continuing recovery, but her other corroborating medical documentation also enables us to reach this conclusion without doubt.

Mrs. Kendall is no longer an isolated, unusual case. As of this writing, I have seen approximately one hundred women with SAD. Many of her complaints have been echoed over and over again by hundreds, if not thousands, of women with similar symptoms reflecting the ravaging effects of silicone-associated disease.

As an allergist/immunologist, I have seen the multifaceted characteristics of this illness. Having dealt with allergic/immunologic reactions to substances over the years and published a paper on how Lupus can have essentially the same symptoms as an allergy to penicillin, I have come to the conclusion that drugs and chemicals may cause many types of unusual and severe allergic reactions.

For example, penicillin can produce hives, rashes, serum sickness, fevers and false blood tests. Thus, a single substance can produce many different reactions through various mechanisms in the human body. This is what I believe is the case with silicone. Some people can tolerate silicone well, just as some people never become allergic to penicillin, no matter how much they receive. Others may receive only a few doses of penicillin and have a life-threatening, or even fatal, reaction. A single substance can cause a multitude of problems in different people at different times. This is what I believe is the spectrum of silicone-associated disease.

I have the utmost faith that Pamela Kendall will continue to improve and lead a normal life at last. I know her book will give hope, faith and courage to many other women and men who may be suffering from silicone-associated disease.

# 1

## THE ALTERATION

Looking back on that fateful time, it all appears to have been merely a bad dream. Surely, I had thought, after awakening the nightmare would end. Sadly, I was not asleep. How did I live through it? Perhaps I prevailed by simply not knowing the torturous path that lay ahead.

Although one rarely has everything, I was quite fortunate to lead a rather charmed life. As a child, I grew up on a plantation in the Mississippi delta and was blessed with many advantages. In my later teen years, I traveled extensively with my family and lived in countries throughout South America, Europe and Africa; I received my formal education in London, Paris and Geneva. However, I also had my share of misfortune along the way.

A near fatal automobile accident in my teens left me critically injured and required months of recuperation. It was a miracle that I survived. An off-duty paramedic happened upon the wreckage and administered CPR. If he had not, I would certainly have died on the spot. My recovery, though, was a painful lesson in patience— a lesson to be repeated many times during the course of my life.

# TORN ILLUSIONS

Following this early brush with mortality, a failing marriage at a young age ended in divorce. My South African husband had been miserably unhappy in the United States, and I was unable to live in Johannesburg so far removed from my own culture. After the birth of my second child in South Africa, I faced a most difficult decision. My marriage had crumbled beyond repair. Aside from the tensions caused by our incompatible backgrounds, my young husband found it difficult to accept the responsibilities of a wife and two children. Nonetheless, I considered a South African divorce to be out of the question. I would have been allowed custody, but rigid domestic laws prevented me from ever leaving the country with my children. Despite this, we managed to get out. Although I regretted the resulting separation from their father, I returned to the United States with my children Carl, a three-and-a-half year old toddler, and Deborah, a six-month old infant, to file for a divorce.

I rented a small house near my grandmother and sister and opened a nursery school as a means of support. In this way, I was able to earn an income while still being able to care for my children. Their father had not furnished — nor did I request—financial assistance. Once we were settled back in the United States we existed on a very restricted budget, but I learned self-sufficiency during this healing period as I waited for my divorce to be finalized.

A year later, Carl, Deborah and I left for London, where my mother and father resided. I worked with my father at his oil brokerage company and eventually began dating the man who would become my future husband, Paul Kendall. I was initially attracted to Paul's maturity, as opposed to the youthful irresponsibility of my first husband. Paul was also intelligent, handsome and entertaining. Foremost, he loved children.

Eventually, Paul, the former president of Conoco Europe, moved to Florida, where he had other business interests. The children and I joined him there and we were married. We bought a beautiful old, stucco oceanfront house on the exclusive Hillsboro Mile just north of Fort Lauderdale, and I undertook with pleasure its renovation and decoration. Having now established firm roots, I imagined that we would stay in our home on the ocean forever. My life with Paul seemed safe and secure. It wasn't long before we formed and organized three related oil companies. In structuring the corporations, my husband decided that I should be the president of one, Kendall Petroleum. Paul admired my young exuberance and was pleased with my eagerness and abilities.

Though far from a perfect husband, Paul was a wonderful father, which was very important to me. He adored my children, and delighted in their activities, birthday parties and school functions. By now, Carl was eight, and Deborah was five.

I had a large house to keep up, and I also had to run a business. Needing an extra pair of helping hands, we hired a young woman, Teresa St. Forte from the Virgin Islands, who came to live with us. Teresa remained for a long time, becoming not only a helpmate, but a trusted and valued friend. Without her support I might not have survived the years to come.

My family and I lived quite a glamorous life. We had many friends, socialized frequently and entertained often. I enjoyed cooking and took pleasure in preparing for our numerous parties. My world was busy and exciting between work-related trips and family vacations, which included island cruises on our yacht, *Red Magic.* Above all, I had good health, energy and vitality. In order to take proper care of my family, I painstakingly planned our meals, shopped in health food stores and even ordered monthly home deliveries of spring water. Exercise was an integral part of my daily routine: beach walks, bike rides and morning aerobics. It was a very good time in my life. I held great expectations for the future.

During these years, plastic surgery had become the rage. Many women, over coffee, openly acknowledged their surgery and casually revealed the details of their cosmetic alterations. Plastic surgery was readily available— and not only for the wealthy. Women of poor means would put aside some money from their paychecks for their upcoming operations. The media emphasis on youth, fitness and beauty encouraged the trend; women of all ages became willing participants. And why not? Many perceived the expense, along with any discomfort or inconvenience incurred, to be a small price to pay for the look of beauty and youth. Outwardly, the rewards appeared to be great.

I prefer to think the reason I decided to have a breast implantation was reconstructive. Although I had a C-cup measurement, I also had a lot of excessively loose and sagging skin as a result of nursing both my children for long periods. Having remarried, I wanted to be more beautiful for my new, handsome and successful husband. So, during 1980, I consulted a plastic surgeon. He told me that I was a good candidate for breast implants, or, as he called it, augmentation mammaplasty. I felt the implants would increase my attractiveness as well as correct and repair the post-lactation breast trauma. I enthusiastically agreed to it. Of course, I never read the package insert on the implants. Even if I did, realistically, a review of the information available at that point would not have changed my decision. Manufacturers did not supply warnings of the potential dangers of this type of surgery. Before undergoing it, I did question my gynecologist, Dr. Gregory Zann, about the safety of silicone breast implants and asked if my own implantation was prudent. Dr. Zann said it was an excellent idea.

The surgery was performed in October. It was to be a "minor surgical procedure" that several million other women around the world had also undergone. It was a seemingly inconsequential act, but it would irrevocably alter my future. At first this seemed to be a change for the better. In a matter of a few short hours, my illusions became reality. Looking into the mirror, I was delighted by "the new me."

Unfortunately, the problems began from Day One. Though I told no one about it, I was besieged by what appeared to be a variety of strange symptoms and pain. They continued during the next weeks. Over the Thanksgiving holiday, while we were vacationing in Aspen, Colorado, I confessed to Paul that I had not felt entirely well since the date of my surgery

"Perhaps," I said, "I contracted a virus in the hospital."

He looked at me strangely, but I hardly took notice.

Feeling poorly and leery of damaging my recent surgery by an accidental fall, I did not ski at all during the trip.

# TORN ILLUSIONS

During the months that followed, I experienced more intense pain, predominantly on the left side. This agony continued into the new year when, in addition, I began feeling a sharp, piercing pain with both a squeezing and pulling sensation in the left breast. When this lasted, I became worried that the implant had become dislodged. I telephoned my plastic surgeon's office. The nurse informed me that it was a normal occurrence and would subside. Without giving me further explanation, she said that an office visit was not necessary and hung up.

Over the next few months the pain did not subside and recurring allergic as well as flu-like symptoms began. At first, they were mild, but gradually they intensified and increased in number. I complained to my family physician of a sore throat, nausea and aches in my arms and legs. There were swollen glands under my arms, in my neck and throat and behind my ears. I often had headaches, chills and low grade fevers of 99 to 101 degrees. Daily antihistamines did not relieve the nasal stuffiness and itching or the sporadic rashes which occurred on various areas of my body. Although these symptoms began after my implantation, no one questioned the possibility of a correlation between the surgery and the illness, now set in motion.

In the summer of that year, I started developing additional problems. Now I had constant abdominal and lower back pain. When it continued, Dr. Zann examined me and suggested that it could be endometriosis. After trying other remedies, he recommended a hysterectomy without the removal of my ovaries. Although I was only in my early thirties, and the thought of having a hysterectomy at such a young age was very troubling, I was grateful for the two beautiful, healthy children I already had. Since I now was wracked by continuous pain and willing to do anything to feel better, I consented. The pathology report after the operation seemed to confirm Dr. Zann's diagnosis since endometriosis was found to be present. Afterward, I waited for relief; however, my abdominal pain persisted. I reported it to Dr. Zann, "I'm sorry to say the operation has not stopped my pain." In fact, by the fall, my symptoms had advanced and horribly progressed.

# TORN ILLUSIONS

On a Sunday morning in October 1981, I awoke feeling acutely ill; my face was red and terribly swollen. I had wracking chills and debilitating fever. Frightened, I telephoned my general practitioner's office. He told me to go to the emergency room of the hospital.

"A physician-on-call will meet you in the emergency room and conduct laboratory tests." The test results were inconclusive. Other doctors were called in. There still was no diagnosis, but the doctors suspected that an autoimmune illness called lupus might be responsible for my severe symptoms. By this time I was nearly at my wit's end.

After that distressing episode, my health continued to decline. My legs were stiff and I developed severe headaches, accompanied by frightening periods of memory loss. The doctors still didn't know what was wrong with me. I was still without a diagnosis. When I developed pancreatitis, my mother urged me to make an appointment at Oscher Clinic. My husband Paul approved of the consultation; so we traveled to New Orleans together and checked into the visitors' annex adjoining the clinic. However, my husband, whose displeasure with my illness mounted every day, quickly excused himself and departed. I felt completely abandoned.

I had counted on Paul's support during my medical review at the clinic; instead, I found myself alone. Sick, exhausted, with barely the strength to walk, I tried to manage the strenuous daily physicians' appointments and testing on my own. It was very difficult, but I wanted to know what was wrong and, more than anything, I wanted to get well. During one examination, I saw an endocrinologist, Dr. Locke, who diagnosed a mumps-like viral infection due to the evidence of several gland enlargements (including the parotid jaw gland) and an inflamed pancreas. Dr. Locke further noted my lapses in memory and the perplexing "rashes" on my stomach and legs. He diagnosed these as purpuras. (I would later learn that this particular skin eruption is associated with inflammation, vascular abnormalities and drug reactions.) A clinic immunologist volunteered another possible diagnosis. He felt I could have a connective-tissue disease. All

# TORN ILLUSIONS

these illnesses, attacking me one after another, only increased my feelings of discouragement.

Nevertheless, Dr. Locke assured me that I would, indeed, recover. He advised that, upon my return home, I seek out an infectious disease specialist.

I called Dr. Zann, my gynecologist, who referred me to Dr. David Droller. Infectious diseases were his speciality. Dr. Droller began my examination by ordering viral studies. They came back negative and supplied no clues. All the while, I grew steadily worse. At one point, when I collapsed at home, with my head pounding and my body quivering uncontrollably, Teresa had to call 911. My children, who were returning from a shopping trip with a family friend, watched fearfully as paramedics carried me into the ambulance and took me to the hospital.

Lying in the hospital bed, my body in pain, my mind in turmoil, I worried first about one thing, then another: my health, my finances and, most of all, my poor children. Their agonized faces as they had watched me being placed in the ambulance haunted me. That evening, as I looked out the window, the phone suddenly rang. It was Carl, my twelve-year-old son. He told me in a trembling voice that he had injured himself playing on our boat dock. Badly bleeding from a large gash on his leg, he'd been rushed to the emergency room by my husband who, fortunately, was home when the accident occurred.

"Mom," Carl said, "why can't you be here now? You've always been there for me. I need you so much."

As tears ran down my cheeks, I tried to reassure him.

"Dearest, you know how much I love you. I'd give anything to be with you, but," my voice broke, "I can't. I'm just too sick." Never had I felt so much despair. I tried to go on.

"You know Paul will take good care of you, and I'll be home as soon as I possibly can." My words sounded empty even to me. I knew, to a hurt, frightened boy of twelve, afraid and lonely in the emergency room of a hospital, such words were meaningless anyway. What really mattered to him—no matter what her excuse—was that his mother wasn't there. It felt like desertion. His unanswered need was something that, despite his pity and love for me, neither of us could ever erase. We both would carry with us always.

But it was to be one of many, many occasions when I could not function as their mother, and the sadrness, hopelessness, and disappointment I felt were always the same.

Nevertheless, though I felt miserable, there was nothing I could do. Helplessly, I looked down at my wracked body. Trying to rise on my elbow, I succumbed my own dizzying weakness and fell back. I promised myself I'd be well and able to tend to my children's needs very soon.

Yet the horror of my illness went on. By this time, Dr. Droller had diagnosed encephalopathy (an unspecified brain disorder of unknown causation). He realized that I had a serious and bewildering illness. Day by day, I felt my once-active life collapsing all around me. I now began to fear becoming an invalid.

Distressed, Dr. Droller consulted his former professor, Dr. Jay Sanders, an immunologist at the University of Miami. For a short time, they gave me doses of gamma globulin. Then Dr. Sanders discovered that my family physician, Dr. Arthur Naddell, had given me monthly injections of gamma globulin to boost my immune system. After learning this, Dr. Sanders believed that my immune system had produced antibodies to the foreign proteins in the gamma globulin, which thereby produced an autoimmune-like condition. As a result, my crippled immune system could not handle the viral infection. (It was later theorized that, in my case, the gamma globulin treatments may have contributed to the burden of my body's overstimulated immune system, then engaged in warfare with silicone.) Dr. Sanders warned Dr. Droller, "Another injection of gamma globulin might kill her."

In fact, I already felt close to death. I could not know it was to be only one of many times.

They halted the shots, but still no one had come to a final diagnosis of what was wrong with me.

In the fall, I entered my second year after having had the silicone implantation. I was now completely incapacitated and bedridden. No one knew why. No one knew when I would be well again. The doctors felt I needed a lengthy recuperation. Under such circumstances, they knew my marriage might be greatly strained. Dr. Sanders offered to speak to my husband.

On the day that Dr. Sanders discussed my injection-associated serum sickness with Paul and told my husband that he predicted a recovery would take months, my husband's simmering resentment boiled over. He became furious and said he could not accept my debilitating illness. The doctor's reassurances did nothing to quell his fury. Listening to their loud voices, lying in our bedroom alone and seriously ill, I knew that Paul felt he had not only lost his social companion, but the person who kept his house in order and was his business partner, as well. All the responsibilities of cooking, housekeeping and chauffeuring of the children, which I previously assumed, now fell completely on Teresa's shoulders. Eventually, as my condition worsened and Teresa's duties increased, Paul hired another employee, Viergela, to lift some of the burden from Teresa.

By then, Paul was continuously resentful about how long I was taking to get well and how miserable his own life was because of it. However, his bitterness did not hold a candle to mine. Not only had the husband I loved become a stranger, and the job I'd once enjoyed so much been taken away, but, more importantly, I helplessly watched as, one by one, my pleasures and responsibilities as a mother also ended. First, it was the more mundane things—cooking, housekeeping and the taxiing of the children which fell on Teresa's shoulders. Then, while I was trying to adjust to the loss of these things because of my invalid state, it suddenly struck me that I was beginning to lose much more.

The realization came about two weeks before my daughter's tenth birthday.

Children, as you probably have also observed, have a boundless optimism, which we adults lose as we mature and adjust to reality. Nowhere is their optimism and our pessimism more apparent than right before birthdays and holidays.

So, even though by this time I felt I had been ill forever and my once bright hopes for recovery were fading, to Deborah, my darling nine-year-old daughter, my recovery was just around the corner. That meant I would certainly be well before her tenth birthday.

On that Tuesday, she burst into my room with incredible energy and a glowing look.

"Mom, Mom," she called. "It's time to discuss my party this year. Remember you promised when you were sick at Christmastime anything I wanted to do we would."

Perhaps it was because her words were coming so quickly, or perhaps it was that watching her, Debbie's enthusiasm reignited my own. I allowed her to go on for several minutes, and I enjoyed her spirit in spite of myself. Then reality set in.

Propping myself on an elbow, I lifted my head up from the bed. I sighed. What I had been hiding, even from myself, confronted me. I was too weak to handle the large festivities at a child's party. My frustration was limitless. I had always enjoyed giving the children wonderful birthdays with all their friends present. Now I was so incapacitated that not only could I not make the preparations, I could not even attend. Debbie and I would not share confidences as we happily went to the store to choose the perfect outfit for her. She would not stand near me to sample the splendid cake I was baking nor "bug me" to find out what her big present was. This year I would not even be able to choose one myself.

I gently tried to explain how weak I was, and that this year she and a few friends would have to go to lunch and a movie with Teresa. The tears in her eyes told me how very disappointed she was. Of course, I was too. Debbie would never have another tenth birthday, nor the party at which we both wanted to celebrate it.

As I swallowed my own bitter tears, I wondered how many other special occasions we would miss. Luckily we did not know.

At this time, having rejected Dr. Sander's prognosis, Paul arranged an evaluation for me at the Mayo Clinic. He hoped to obtain a more decisive diagnosis and thus hasten my recovery. At Paul's insistence, we traveled to Rochester, Minnesota, in the dead of winter. By then, I had become so weak that he asked a family member for the use of a corporate jet. Once there, I was admitted to the clinic's hospital as an in-patient due to my degenerating condition. The Mayo physicians began a two-day review of my medical records. Paul became restless. At the end of the second day, he suddenly called off the examination in progress and curtly informed me that he intended to leave. Too ill to be left alone in Minnesota or to get home without his aid, I accompanied Paul on the return trip to Florida.

Within a few weeks, a letter arrived from my treating physician at the Mayo Clinic. The doctor, an infectious disease specialist, attributed my illness to a protracted viral infection, despite a lack of proof indicating a virus to be the causative agent. Discouraged, I began feeling that none of my doctors really understood the exact nature of my illness.

I felt more reassured when I learned that my family's London physician, Dr. John Ind, planned to come to the United States in the spring. Surely, I thought, he knew me so well he would detect what was the matter. He said he would visit us in Florida. When he arrived and examined me, I asked him for his opinion of my ill health. He agreed with Dr. Sander's theory that my immune system was not functioning normally. Hoping to raise my spirits, he complimented me on my fortitude in coping with my illness. "However, I'm very concerned about your husband's unsupportive, if not detrimental, attitude," he added. Dr. Ind made every effort, as had other physicians, to convince Paul that I would eventually recover. It was to no avail.

My life continued to go down hill. My health did not improve, and I could no longer be consoled by more promises of recovery as no one could tell me definitively how long it would take or why my immune system had gone awry. Adding to my uneasiness, the AIDS epidemic was becoming public at this time and I was worried about the effect of the shots I had taken. Fortunately, due to the method used in preparation, gamma globulin was not a contaminated blood product. (Doctors later conclusively ruled out the existence of the AIDS virus by immune system testing.)

Through the fog of perpetual illness, as the days turned into weeks and the months became years, I grew more concerned that my doctors had either missed or overlooked the real diagnosis. "I feel poisoned," I told them. "Clearly, my symptoms developed after the implantation," and I asked each of my physicians about a cause-effect association. It was impossible to miss their amused looks when I suggested this possibility.

By then, I was noticing that my left implant looked different, not as full as the right one. I brought this to the attention of Dr. Droller, who also noted their lack of symmetry and suggested it might be due to silicone leakage. Concerned, he contacted the plastic surgeon who performed my implantation and scheduled a consultation for me.

In his office, the surgeon examined me and gave me a mammogram. "The implants appear to be normal," he said somewhat relieved. After that examination, the question of silicone leakage, first posed by Dr. Droller, was no longer pursued, nor was the possibility that my implants were related to my sickness.

Nevertheless, my health declined precipitously. During my second year after the implantation, I left the house only for doctor visits. My enforced confinement led to greater isolation. I had no family living nearby, and most of my friends and acquaintances soon lost interest in a chronically ill person. Only Teresa and two other friends were steadfast in offering me the encouragement I needed to lift my spirits and to help me maintain a positive attitude in spite of my failing health and faltering marriage. These three companions and my children were my link to the outside world. They waited for the restoration of my health and stood by me as my marital situation worsened.

Paul's resentment had grown to the point of alienation. By the following summer, he had dissolved our joint corporations. Next, he moved into a guest-room downstairs. Soon, he began pressuring me to vacate the house and relinquish our property. He often threatened to send me to a nursing facility if I did not go to my mother's of my own accord. As more time passed, and I seemed to be getting worse rather than better, his verbal taunting increased, as did his demands for me to leave. Teresa stayed by my side as often as possible, hoping that her presence would soften his verbal assaults.

Finally, realizing I was in urgent need of legal advice, I telephoned Bruno Di Giulian, a respected divorce attorney. He came to my home for the consultation, not wanting to subject me, in my weakened condition, to a grueling office conference. Lying in my bed,

# TORN ILLUSIONS

weak and discouraged, I tried to explain to him how much I wanted to save my marriage. After hearing how Paul had been acting, he looked saddened and shook his head. As I entered my third year after the silicone implants, I had little choice except to prepare for the separation that Mr. Di Giulian deemed inevitable.

In late fall, despite my heavy heart, I made a determined effort to arrange for the children's Christmas. In an effort to appease Paul's impatience with me and my illness, as I still kept the futile hope our marriage could be salvaged, I also tried to go out socially. I still wanted to please my husband. However, to do this, because I was so ill, I relied on Teresa's assistance. She helped me dress, helped me walk to the car, then drove me to our destinations. During this struggle, I kept reassuring Paul that the critical stage of my illness was passing.

On what was to be my first night out with my husband, I felt as excited as I had when we began dating. I tried to rise from the bed but my body shook as Teresa helped me make up and dress.

"Oh, look," I cried disappointedly, as I put on a creamy blue cashmere sweater and skirt. "I've grown so thin there could be two of me in here. He'll think I'm ugly, and I wanted to be beautiful tonight."

Teresa patted my shoulder and said gently, "He'll know how much effort all this took and he'll be proud of you, just as I am."

"Teresa, you always lift my spirits," I said and smiled.

"That's part of my job," she smiled back. She guided me down the stairs and into the living room where Paul sat waiting on the couch. He jumped to his feet with camera ready, and snapped a photograph of me as we entered the room.

"Paul," I said, surprised, "you've, never taken home pictures before."

A pained look came on his face. "Well, there's always a first time." He reddened and added, "Anyway, it's a memorable occasion, isn't it?"

"Of course," I murmured, "that's a sweet thought."

Still, I couldn't help thinking his behavior and obvious embarrassment were strange, but little did I know that one day that very photograph would be offered as a proof that his wife was ambulatory in order for my husband to file for divorce.

That night, I put the incident out of my mind. Paul had insisted we go out to dinner with another couple at the yacht club where we were members. Despite my shakiness, I forced myself to hold up through the meal and small talk, though my head was swimming and my arm so weak that I could barely lift my fork.

With pure will I made it though the night and even allowed myself to believe that my illness was drawing to a close. It was another futile hope. I soon learned that this wasn't so. My immunologist explained that some immune system illnesses have up and down periods, but I felt that the "up" period was, in large part, due to my stubborn nature and my desperate desire to be well. Although activity aggravated my symptoms, I forced myself to get up each day, only to fall back down again. Finally, I began thinking that I might be fighting a losing battle.

Despite all my efforts to forestall a final break, my marriage ended two weeks before Christmas, when Paul left without warning. Our plans to have a quiet holiday with the children and Teresa at the Ocean Reef Club in Key Largo were canceled. I had anticipated that a family vacation would mollify Paul's resentment and frustration over my health problems and provide some time in an environment we all had always enjoyed. However, my husband chose to spend the season in Aspen, Colorado.

Shortly thereafter, his attorney telephoned to notify me of Paul's intention to obtain a divorce. My husband was adamant in his desire to break free from a marriage that bound him to an invalid wife. I not only had to deal with my children's disappointments about Paul's absence on Christmas Day, but I also had to come to terms with his abandonment.

In order that Carl and Deborah would still enjoy the holiday, I sent them to The Ocean Reef Club with a dependable friend, Wendy Germi, and her two children. I remained at home with Teresa to handle the attorneys and Paul's demands. Although I pleaded for a legal separation to gain time, hoping we could resolve our differences, Paul insisted on a divorce, offering me increasing sums of money.

## TORN ILLUSIONS

Needing peace, and physically too weak to bear the stress of a courtroom confrontation, I had no other option but to sign the divorce settlement paper his attorney sent mine. The terms of the contract allowed me one more year before I had to vacate the house in which my children and I lived. This final desertion by my husband and the anticipated loss of my home were crushing blows and today are still hurtful memories.

Nevertheless, I willed myself to go on and to get better as soon as I possibly could. However, I misjudged the seriousness of my health situation and mistakenly expected to bounce back from all my adversities if only quiet could be restored to my household. I was wrong. It would take much more than serenity for me to recover.

Despite my sorrow at the divorce and my growing health problems, Carl and Deborah were now my primary concern. Their anguish over the traumatic loss of their stepfather was compounded by the uncertainty about their mother's health. Many times I felt like giving up. What kept me going was the need to establish some sense of security for my children.

# 2

## DISCOVERY

Over the following year, my illness continued. Sometimes I felt better, sometimes worse. Soon the time came for my children, Teresa and I to leave our Hillsboro Beach home. Although I had little physical stamina and was constantly fighting fatigue, I carefully paced myself and gathered enough energy to find and lease an apartment. I could not even think of undertaking a taxing search for a permanent home. My doctors were no longer looking for an explanation for my medical problems, and, as another year went by, I tried to ignore and deny the array of chronic symptoms which besieged me. By then, I had almost forgotten what it felt like to enjoy normal health.

In spite of my health problems, I still believed myself to be on the mend and thought that ultimately, I would recover completely. A physician had once told me that if a patient did not die in the absence of diagnosis and treatment, or spontaneously recover, a cause of illness always surfaced eventually. I lived with this hope and waited with unfounded optimism. Perhaps it was a blessing that I did not have the gift of precognition.

## TORN ILLUSIONS

Another blow struck in the summer of 1984. Teresa and I noticed a slight chemical odor in my clothing. We were at a loss to determine its origin as Teresa never used bleach and used only mild detergents when laundering clothes. When I told Dr. Droller about it, he was equally baffled and suggested a change in laundry products. Although we tried various detergents at home, the odor in my clothing continued, growing even more disconcerting. At the same time, I developed breathing difficulties. Dr. Droller prescribed antibiotics, but my respiratory symptoms continued to worsen. One problem followed another. Soon, I developed dry eye syndrome. I went to see Dr. Nelson Redfern, an ophthalmologist. He administered the Schirmer eye test. It revealed an immune-related disorder which was irreversible. Daily, I was getting excruciating headaches followed by dizzy spells. The nagging pain in my upper-left abdominal area grew worse and my allergic reactions to environmental chemicals increased.

By the fall, on the threshold of my fifth year after the implants, the chemical odor in the upper body areas of my clothing had become very pungent. Though Teresa tried, washing the clothes vigorously would not remove the odor. Then I began having night sweats. To my horror, they bleached the color out of my bed linens. Teresa was alarmed, and I was totally devastated. I felt completely defeated and despondent over the development of this new and horrifying symptom.

As the chemical stench intensified, I became even more terrified about the eventual outcome of my disease. I began to feel that I was about to die.

Neither were my children spared. They were eyewitnesses to the personal horror growing in my life. Daily, they watched Teresa removing reeking, stained clothes and linens from my bedroom. Many of them had to be thrown away in the trash.

I saw the growing fear in their eyes as they tiptoed into my room each day after school, seeing the dark lines beneath my eyes grow deeper, the deathly pallor of my skin become more waxy, as I grew weaker and thinner. They, too, wondered if I would die. Lying propped up with pillows to aid my breathing, I fought for every breath when speaking to them.

Despite my fervent desire to remain part of my children's lives, noise, even music, began to agitate me. Though they didn't complain, gradually Carl and Deborah invited fewer friends over to the apartment, soon none. How could they explain my condition to friends their own age when neither they, I, nor even my physicians understood it? I felt I was becoming an embarrassment to my children rather than a mother to be relied upon. This left me even more dejected.

As daily my condition worsened, Teresa, seeing my own inability to act, took charge and drove me to see Dr. Sanders. There were tears in my eyes as we sat together in his office and I told him of my experiences. A startled Dr. Sanders was apologetic.

"Oh, my God. I'm so sorry," he exclaimed.

He sat silent and pensive for a few moments, then blurted out, "You've been chemically poisoned!"

Hearing his words should have added to my alarm, but I was flooded with relief. To have received, after all this time, an explanation of any sort, if only a partial one, made me feel better. I felt it an important step toward finally getting a diagnosis of what was really wrong with me.

Since Dr. Sanders was no longer in private practice, he referred me to Dr. Ira Finegold, an allergy and immunology specialist. I made an immediate appointment. When we went for the consultation, Teresa and I brought along several articles of my clothing and bed linen for the doctor to examine. Noting both the odor and the bleaching of the fabrics, Dr. Finegold also suspected chemical poisoning. Now he sought to identify the cause of this reaction. The doctor instructed Teresa to sort through and discard all the chemical products and substances that I used on a daily basis. We did. However, this was to no avail, as the chemical odor, which was concentrated in the front and back chest areas of my clothing, persisted. It was not until we noticed, one day, that my breast pain and discomfort radically worsened at the same time as the odor, that our attention again focused on the implants.

Not long afterward, during an office examination, redness and swelling developed under my arm when Dr. Finegold pressed on the prostheses. Even with this indication of implant involvement, I could not have known that silicone poisoning was the actual cause of my illness. Dr. Finegold and I lacked tangible, corroborative evidence. Nevertheless, I felt hope; the possibility of a diagnosis meant the possibility of treatment. This strengthened my determination to conquer the illness.

Finegold next decided to test my skin with silicone. The first patch test he gave me was with a commercial grade of silicone. It produced a positive reaction consisting of welts and redness. Because of this result, Dr. Finegold did a more discriminating test using a purer grade of silicone. He spoke to Dr. Diran Seropian, the plastic surgeon who performed my implant surgery, and asked from where the prosthesis he had inserted in my chest had come. Then he contacted the manufacturer, who subsequently supplied us with an implant identical to my own. Once he had the prosthesis, Dr. Finegold repeated the procedure. He conducted the second patch test with the same Dow Corning/Heyer-Shulte gel that my implants contained. He selected four items and numbered them: the silicone gel, the implant shell, nickel sulfate and benzocaine. Then Dr. Finegold tested my reactions to the last two substances, because they are common allergy-producing contactants. He didn't tell me the number sequence he employed during the testing. He described it as "blind" skin-testing. The shell, nickel and benzocaine patch tests proved negative, but the silicone gel produced two red, raised positive reactions. It was in this manner that my allergy to silicone was conclusively determined. Two years later, a skin test of pure, medical-grade silicone, injected under the skin of my forearm, produced another allergic reaction. It consisted of redness, swelling, welts and rashes. Because of the harsh reaction I had, the doctors decided the substance had to be surgically removed.[1]

When conducting the second allergy testing, Dr. Finegold came across an article in the medical literature regarding silicone and the immune system. While I was with him, he telephoned the author, Dr. Habal, and they discussed my positive reaction to the silicone.[2]

They also discussed the implant's capability to "bleed" silicone-gel. In spite of having lived through five years with silicone implantations, I had not heard of the possibility of routine silicone leakage through an intact shell until that moment. It was another frightening possibility.

After gaining new insights from Dr. Habal, Dr. Finegold ordered a second mammogram. It revealed my left implant had more laxity and shallow folds than the one on the right. This test showed a change from my earlier mammogram. It indicated a loss or "bleed" of silicone. Because of the findings of both the mammogram and the skin test, Dr. Finegold said, "I have no other alternative but to recommend the removal of your implants." At the time, however, he was not completely convinced of silicone's responsibility for my overall illness. In 1985 these were uncharted waters. It was only later that compelling medical findings, documentation, events and the course of my illness would lead him to the final conclusion: silicone, from the day of my implantation, had been the sole cause of my medical problems.

My symptoms had rapidly accelerated during the preceding months. Therefore, Dr. Finegold decided that the surgery to remove my implants had to be done as soon as possible. I was now suffering attacks of pain in the upper-left part of my abdomen. These became more and more severe and were accompanied by a peculiar burning sensation in this area. The dizziness I felt was unrelenting, my ears rang, and my eye problems worsened. My arms and legs tingled and felt numb.

Unfortunately, however, Dr. Finegold's plan to proceed immediately were halted when a late-night telephone call on August 19th brought the shocking news of my father's unexpected death. My parents lived in Singapore, but traveled twice a year for one month at a time to the United States, where they maintained another home. My daughter had been vacationing with them and was standing at my father's side when he was stricken by a rupture of the aorta, which instantly took his life. Regardless of how ill I was, I wanted to be there with my mother and daughter. My son and I hurriedly prepared for the funeral. Our flight arrived early the next morning. We rented a car and then Carl drove nearly three hours to reach my parents' house in the country. Completely dazed by the announcement about my father, worried over the result of my daughter seeing her grandfather die and physically ill as well, I was thankful for both my son's presence and supportive strength. Braced by his steady arm, I managed the walk down the church aisle at the funeral service. I returned to Florida with my children a week later, shaken by grief.

The following month another issue faced us. My son's social activities, now that he could drive, overtook his interest in school grades. Although he and I talked and talked about his falling grades, I was too ill to give him the supervision a sweet but rambunctious teenager required. Finally, I decided we had to confront the issue. One afternoon, I gathered what little strength I had and, that evening, told him we needed to speak seriously.

"Carl, " I said, "we've all been through a lot and you're a wonderful help to me."

He broke in. "Mom, I want to do even more."

I nodded. "But," I said in a trembling voice, "these should be very special years of preparation in your life and," I bit my lip to hold back my tears, "you see how ill I am. There's no way I can share or teach you the things I should." I looked sadly at him. "Carl, I've decided it's best for you to go to boarding school near your Grandmother's. With Grandfather dead, you'll be a comfort to her, and," I stumbled over the next words, "it will be better for you, for your future, if you are in a good school."

His face crestfallen, he didn't even try to argue. He just nodded.

"If you think it's best."

"Yes," I murmured. "I really do."

A week later, as I watched him leave, my heart was heavy. I thought about all the special moments in his life that would now be taken away from me and, when the door closed and he could no longer hear me, I cried for us both.

That next week, I developed a new complication—a daily fever. This further complicated plans to schedule the removal of the implants. Laboratory tests were needed in order to rule out the possibility of infection. Once the tests were run, Dr. Finegold assessed the fever to be an inflammatory response to the implants. As I waited for the plans for the operation to be completed, I began feeling even weaker. I felt that my time was running out, and spoke to Dr. Finegold of my concern. Once again he tried to reassure me but I could sense his distress.

Prophetically, a short time afterward, I began having periods of involuntary trembling, shaking, and jerking. When I told the doctor he had me immediately admitted to the hospital, where they were termed "siezure-like episodes." Years later, discovered the results of an electroencephalogram (EEG) subsequently conducted by neurologist Dr. Maria-Carmen Wilson of the University of South Florida School of Medicine. It showed seizure activity on the right side of my brain, which confirmed that these "episodes" had actually been true seizures.

In the future, there would be testimony involving other women with comparable, implant-related neurological involvement. Their resulting documented deaths would be established by the testimony of Dr. Bernard Patten, a neurologist at Baylor University Hospital, who testified before the 1992 FDA panel review.[3]

However, at that time we knew little. Dr. Finegold decided the best course was to push ahead on having the implants removed. He contacted Dr. Seropian, who would perform the surgery. Seropian had earlier concurred that, given the circumstances of allergy and toxicity, the explanation—though quite unusual—was in order. In discussing the details of my projected surgery, Dr. Finegold requested that the fibrous capsule surrounding the implants, and any adjacent tissue which was contaminated, be excised as well. Since I was too weak to tolerate a general anesthesia, Dr. Finegold decided this would have to be accomplished under local anesthetic. During the surgery my head would be elevated to lessen the dizziness, which had intensified to such a degree that it became overpowering when I lay flat. The arrangements for surgery also included transferring me to Broward General Hospital, where Dr. Seropian was Chief of Staff.

The morning I was to leave for Broward, Dr. Finegold stopped by my room before signing my release. Aware of how fearful I was about undergoing the operation in my weakened condition, he tried to uplift my spirits but seemed rather preoccupied himself. His face brightened, however, when, through the window, the vision of a brilliant rainbow caught his eye.

"Look!" He said, motioning toward the sky. "That's a good omen for you. You're going to be all right."

The operation was performed almost five years to the day of my original silicone implant surgery. Though there was a strong possibility of scarring as a result of this new surgery, it did not seem important during this critical period. Survival outweighed any other consideration. My implantation had almost cost me my life.

As things turned out, I was fortunate. Not only was the surgery successful, but there were no visible traces of scarring. More importantly, I experienced sudden relief from many of my previous symptoms. The dizziness I had constantly experienced disappeared within hours; my headaches vanished; and some allergic symptoms went away. My head felt clear for the first time in five years; the fevers ceased and chemical sensitivities receded. Some other symptoms disappeared. I was so elated by these positive changes that I expected a speedy, complete recovery. Instead, long years of recuperation were needed before I recovered from the effects and complications of silicone poisoning. It took at least a three-month period following my explantation before I walked as far as the kitchen. It was six months before I was able to hold a pen in my hand and write legibly, and eight months before I walked the distance to the car and was able to drive.

Still, I now seemed to be on the road to recovery. How could I know that there was more trouble ahead? At the end of 1985, I suffered a particularly horrifying day. On my way to the medical library I looked down at my blouse, meaning to straighten it, and gasped. The blouse was becoming soaked with a foul-smelling liquid. Fearing the worst, I rushed to Dr. Finegold's office. After a quick examination, he telephoned the hospital. "Admit Pamela Kendall as an emergency, I'm sending her right over."

Inside the hospital, I could not stand unaided; I could not sign my name, and I could barely speak. Medics brought over a wheel chair and took me to a room.

# TORN ILLUSIONS

Nurses began to undress me. Chemical excretions with a horrible, offensive odor poured from my body. My clothes and bedlinens had to be constantly changed.

In desperation, Dr. Finegold telephoned several toxicologists and other chemical specialists in pursuit of a treatment. They advised him that nothing could be done. Whether I lived or died, my system had to purge the chemical poisons. Any form of treatment might only push me closer to death. Pondering my deteriorating condition and what he had been told, Dr. Finegold asked that I contact my family. Judging from his agonized expression, I realized that after all I'd been through, another silicone related problem threatened my life once again. I called my son, who immediately came home from boarding school.

Despite how badly it looked, again I survived. After several weeks of treatment, though I had ongoing problems, I was finally allowed to go home. I was so weak, however, that my teenage son had to carry me from the car, up the stairs, to our apartment, as I cried with frustration over his terror and my situation.

Today, physicians familiar with silicone illness have become aware that symptoms may not improve for a protracted period following an explantation. I didn't know this at the time of my toxic crisis, nor were there any support groups for implant-injured women that I could call. Laying bedridden at home during the next weeks, totally incapacitated, feeling totally alone, I had all but given up hope of recovery, when, unexpectedly, my health began to improve. To my surprise, this improvement continued, though its progress was painfully slow.

However, it was not a straight path. During the following months and years, further complications would be diagnosed, documented and slowly resolved. I was not in the clear yet.

# 3

# THE ONLY ONE?

Still, there was reason for rejoicing; my recovery had finally begun and slowly it continued into 1986. Both the number and intensity of my symptoms decreased. At the same time, both Dr. Finegold and I observed that I still had some implant-related complications. There was still a chemical odor, and I had attacks of prolonged and often agonizing pain on my left side. As time went on, these increased and appeared to be signs of some form of metabolic involvement. The fat content in the foods that I ate had the effect of heightening both the pain and the odor. Confronted with many unknowns, Dr. Finegold's primary concern was to determine the extent of my remaining problems.

He began his search for scientific clues by sending some of my soiled clothing to be tested by Dr. Don Roach, a biochemist. Dr. Roach was able to verify the presence of an abnormal chemical rancid in odor in the clothing samples. He also detected that an excessive and abnormal amount of lipids, which are fatty chemicals, were being expelled through my skin and into my clothes. These findings suggested that necessary enzymes had been damaged and, consequently, the fat molecules were not being properly broken down. The elevation of lipid peroxide levels in my blood further indicated the development of a dysfunctioning fat metabolism, but the significance of that finding was not understood at that time.

Later, when researching silicone disorders, I interviewed Dr. Pierre Blais, formerly associated with the Canadian Department of National Health and Welfare, who is an authority on the chemical effects and consequences of having breast implants. During our conversation, I learned that silicone is an "oil" molecule which thereby affects and becomes involved in the metabolism of fat. Dr. Blais explained that this was at the root of my problem. Silicone has been found to attract and absorb the lipid (fat) molecules.[1] He described the process by which the liver produces a substance, peroxidase, to break down the fat molecules. Unable to metabolize the silicone, the liver produces more and more peroxidase, resulting in the abnormally high lipid peroxide levels I exhibited.

Several years afterward, I would also discover from medical testimony given before the 1992 FDA panel review, that the body produces hydrogen peroxide when macrophages, which are activated as part of the defense response, surround foreign invaders such as silicone.[2] This lends credence to the probability that both these chemical processes were involved in the toxic chemicals within my system that led to the earlier bleaching of my clothes.

However, in 1986, the only solution to my metabolic problem that anyone could suggest was that I subsist on a very restricted diet. This made it impossible for me to stabilize my weight. I was already down to one hundred pounds and, since no one could predict the duration of my debilitating condition, how much more weight I would lose was uncertain. Aside from demoralizing me, the intensity of the chemical odor in my clothing and other personal articles ruined many of my belongings. At this point, I also developed an intolerance for numerous foods and drugs that had not previously caused me allergic reactions. It would actually require another two years of recuperation before I could begin to tolerate caffeine, aspirin, antibiotics and other drug products. Five years would pass before I was able to include the smallest amounts of fat in my diet.

During these years, as both my recovery and some of my problems continued, I agonized about how much longer I could stand all this. My existence can only be described as exceedingly tedious and trying. I continued to be physically weak and therefore, socially restricted. Any gains in energy were expended caring for the basic needs of my children. I had few friends, no personal life and, of course, could not work. Teresa's help, not to mention her friendship, remained important to me. With an up and down pattern, I slowly wove my way back, living from one series of medical tests to another, never knowing what the future outcome would be nor what condition would surface next.

One of the things I found most disturbing was that there was very little data available relative to the illness from which I was suffering. As I began to feel better, I decided not only for me, but all the other women who had silicone implants either for reconstructive reasons or because they brought society illusions of beauty, I would start my own medical investigation about silicone. It would involve much research on my part, and though my unpredictable health often impeded me, I resolved not to give up. No matter how ill I felt. I studied the testing and sought examinations conducted by countless specialists in various fields of medicine. Dr. Finegold, as anxious as I, arranged the appointments.

At the same time, Dr. Finegold continued searching for a diagnosis of my remaining symptoms and problems. Some time later one of the medical tests I took showed the definite indications of gland and organ involvement. This prompted Dr. Finegold to order an endocrine work-up for me. When laboratory tests produced irregular results that suggested gland dysfunction, I was terrorized by the possibility of having developed a brain tumor. After another series of tests, in agony I waited weeks for the results. Fortunately, subsequent MRI and CAT scans determined that I did not have a tumor. However, the pituitary gland, which is the master gland situated in the brain, and the left adrenal, which produces metabolic hormones, were both shown to be enlarged. Both of these glands are essential for life.

Their enlargements surprised us, since they had been found normal in earlier tests. My prolactin level (a hormone secreted by the pituitary gland that regulates breast milk production) was also elevated. This would not return to normal levels for three years.

I visited Dr. Larry Fishman, an endocrinologist at the University of Miami. He told me that an elevation in the prolactin level can be implant related and the resulting breast leakage that I experienced is prevalent in other women with breast implants.[3] The perpetual stimulation of the vital pituitary gland by these devices is, undoubtedly, unhealthy and potentially harmful, as evidenced by my own pituitary gland enlargement.

A medical journal article published years later associated elevated prolactin levels with autoimmune illness. Although the studies referred to were not implant-related, there seemed to be a relationship.[4] If elevated prolactin levels are involved in autoimmune illness, and if the silicone breast implant does cause an elevation of the prolactin hormone, there may very well be a link when implants produce autoimmune-like disorders. I feel strongly that this warrants medical investigation and study. Women with breast implants should be advised to have their physicians check their prolactin levels, a test easily performed by most commercial laboratories.

By 1988, the doctors' ongoing medical exploration of my condition revealed more significant organ and gland involvement. Therefore, Dr. Finegold worked toward ruling out any underlying abnormality other than silicone poisoning and related illness. In the meantime, my intermittent pain, metabolic irregularities and erratic laboratory test results continued. One metabolic specialist recommended an even stricter food management and elimination program. He suggested that I recheck for Lupus, a diagnostic label which had often been applied to my illness in earlier years. Fortunately, once again the test proved negative.

Then, due to the persistent enlargement of my pancreas, a pancreatic arteriogram was performed. Unexpectedly, it showed a "beaded" appearance within the common hepatic artery. (The "beading" of pure, medical-grade silicone has been cited in medical literature.)[5] Radioisotope scanning followed and showed a "hot spot" in the colon that corresponded to the area radiating pain. Neither upper or lower GI series or a colonoscopy had defined it. Once again I had to undergo surgery, albeit minor this time, and a colon polyp, described as representative of an inflammatory, benign and hyperplastic growth, was removed from this area. Also, I was given new ultrasound tests which showed an unspecified abnormality in my left kidney. The "burning" sensation I felt in my skin (now associated with silicone illness and reported by many implant patients) was located in the same painful areas that were found to be inflamed.

These glaring abnormalities, which were concentrated on my left side, indicated chronic inflammation and explained the unremitting pain I still felt in my upper-left quadrant. They further suggested that there was a substantial amount of gel loss through the "bleed" process because of my defective left implant. Although I had been informed that my implants were intact when they were removed (they had been discarded, a routine practice at that time), silicone would later be detected in many areas of my body tissue.

It would take years before many of the related complications of my illness began to improve. For instance, it took over eight years for the pain to dissipate. MRI and CAT scans did not show a return to normal until much later. During this time, the medical probe into my condition proceeded. Dr. Finegold found evidence of antibodies similer to the Epstein-Barr virus, which indicated a previous mononucleosis infection. He attributed the presence of the antibodies to an illness I had contracted in my twenties. Since I exhibited no viral-related symptoms or recurrences of any kind after my explantation, the doctor concluded that the silicone may have interfered with my immune system to the point of rendering it defenseless against otherwise harmless viruses. This may have added to the severity of the illness I had shortly before the implants were removed. Both prior to having silicone implants and after their removal, I was capable of adequately fighting these viruses. Dr. Finegold's conclusion would later be reinforced by the testimony of Dr. Joseph Bellanti of Georgetown University School of Medicine before an FDA panel review of implant safety. Dr. Bellanti said there was a possibility that silicone might reactivate the latent retroviruses which are currently associated with autoimmune illness.[6]

Hormonal involvement was another area the doctors decided to explore. I had attacks of flushing, abdominal cramping and breathing difficulty which seemed to me to be cyclical in nature. The doctors became suspicious that I was reacting unfavorably to my own ovarian hormones and accordingly tracked the fluctuations in my estrogen and progesterone levels for several months. This testing determined that I invariably experienced these attacks when the hormonal levels peaked. After much deliberation, my physicians felt that they should remove my ovaries. This was not a pleasing prospect at my young age, but the extent of my discomfort made surgical intervention necessary and I agreed to it. The doctors did not think it either advisable or safe to risk general anesthetic as I was still frail and weakened.

The prospect of having major surgery under local anesthetic would be horrifying under normal circumstances, but my situation was much more serious. My past medical experiences added to my feelings of terror; however, more than anything, I wanted to get better. I told myself that recovery had now become a greater challenge and this operation another hurdle to overcome.

During this period my son was graduating from All Saints Boarding School. It was a day to which I had long looked forward. So many of the experiences mothers and growing children share had been denied us. The sadness of these losses would always be part of my life. I tried not to think of that now, but to concentrate instead on the wonderfully exciting day ahead.

It would not only be a milestone in Carl's life, but a marker of survival in mine. I was so grateful to be alive and going to this special celebration. I put up a calendar and began marking off the days just as I knew my son would be doing. Never had I been so happy, but somewhere inside a small voice seemed to be telling me not to count on going too much. I turned the voice off and chalked it up to the pessimism of being ill for so long.

However, my health once again took another rapid, bad turn. New plans for surgery were cemented, and I went into the hospital.

# TORN ILLUSIONS

The operation was more difficult than anticipated and my recovery slower. Just as I had feared, as the day of Carl's graduation drew near, my doctors said I was far too ill to make the trip. With much sadness, I knew I would have to ask my mother to go in my place.

Although, by this time, Carl had grown more self-sufficient and was philosophical, saying we would celebrate later at home in Florida where he had chosen a college to enter in the fall, the bitterness and anger I felt were overwhelming.

So many years had passed. Both my children were becoming mature, separate people. Yet, they and I had lost a formative period of their childhood because of my serious, continuous illness due to silicone poisoning. I often thought about the people and companies whose greed and recklessness I believed had caused so much pain.

By summer's end, plans for my surgery were cemented. The night before my operation, Dr. Droller, while on his rounds, noticed my name on a hospital room door. He came in for a visit and I brought him up-to-date on my medical history. Dr. Droller, a compassionate man, was stunned by my story. He said that I should be considered "a humbling case for physicians," for I had proven the medical profession wrong. We could not have known how wrong.

I underwent the ovarian surgery. This time they could give me little pain medication. Small amounts of Demerol, local injections of Lidocaine, and very minute amounts of epidural Lidocaine made me slightly numb. I was still able to move my legs and was conscious of a great deal of pain. The concerned anesthesiologist held my hand, and I was well aware that Dr. Zann found operating under these conditions almost as horrifying as I. Later, he told me how impressed he was by my fortitude. I know, however, that my composure was not due to bravery; I simply had no other choice.

The operation was a success and my improvement dramatic. I perceived this as good fortune and a pivotal point in resolving the problems of my implantation. My morale was boosted. Unfortunately, once again I was overly optimistic. I was not aware that silicone had already spread through my body and that full recovery would not be easily or quickly achieved. Preoccupied with recovering from surgery, I was relieved to find that I suffered no ill effects from my lack of estrogen. Hormonal therapy would not be needed, which was a relief. My doctors had not thought I would be able to tolerate estrogen treatment at that stage of my recovery, if ever. Later, the discovery of silicone's presence in my ovarian tissue, removed during this operation, established its existence in my damaged reproductive glands.

Throughout these years in which I fought for recovery, my physicians presumed that I was something of a medical phenomena, unique in my adverse reaction to silicone implants. Not possessing the knowledge to contradict them, I accepted their opinions. However, my medical odyssey was, in fact, a result of my doctors' misunderstandings as they looked for a strange or obscure reason to explain my seemingly bizarre silicone reaction. After going through a sinuous maze of medical tests, no such explanations could be found. The medical documentation gathered during my medical journey has provided irrefutable evidence of my silicone-induced illness, although it was then regarded as unimportant. At the time, I thought of myself as only a victim of bad luck, unaware of the reality that I was a victim in the true sense of the word.

In the early years, my optimistic spirit would have immediately revived, but now I had learned that just as we finished solving one problem, another seemed to take its place. This time was no exception. In January of 1988, Dr. Finegold contacted the National Institute of Health (NIH) in Bethesda, Maryland. He arranged a screening at NIH for the purpose of gathering information on my lipid metabolism. I went there and found the NIH physicians well acquainted with puzzling and uncommon illnesses. I expected that a review of my "unusual" silicone reaction would be openly received. On the contrary, there seemed to me to be disinterest in my case history and a reluctance on the part of the NIH physicians to discuss the subject of silicone. My questions were met with hazy answers; my examination consisted of several days of only routine tests, and an appointment with a metabolic specialist was never arranged.

My stay in Bethesda was brief and ended abruptly. I left when my family called to tell me of the brutal death of my fourteen year old nephew, my elder sister's son. He had been killed as he crossed a street in Memphis, Tennessee. I was saddened by my sister's loss and distracted by my need to get to Memphis to comfort her. With all these personal problems, I did not question what I felt was the Institute's indifferent attitude toward my condition.

After making hasty arrangements for my children's travel from Florida to Memphis, I flew to my family's home, accompanied by a younger sister, to face another family tragedy. I visited with my grieving sister until Carl and Deborah had to go back to school, and we returned to Fort Lauderdale.

Later, when I had time to reflect on my stay at the Institute, I felt that the NIH physicians were either unwilling to open the door on the silicone controversy or, at best, not prepared to handle the problem.

Within a matter of months, news reports from around the world relating the first accounts of injuries and illnesses sustained from silicone implants began to make headlines. This information, paired with my realization that I was not "one in a million," as one of my surgeons had early on suggested, provided me confirmation that I was not alone. After all, up to this point, I was still under the impression that I could be the only person experiencing medical problems after having received silicone breast implants.

# 4

---

# AWARENESS

Now I knew that other women had developed illnesses as a result of their breast implantations. At this point, midway into my own agonizing struggle to recover, I questioned the lack of medical knowledge surrounding the use of these frequently implanted devices. I began realizing that there was no doubt many women had experienced the same difficulty as I had in obtaining a diagnosis for their symptoms, especially after having been told that their implants were harmless. I asked myself why all physicians seemed so uninformed.

Meanwhile, my own problems were causing other questions. Dr. Roach, who had earlier tested my clothing samples, was perplexed by my case of silicone poisoning. He began to seek out what had been published in medical literature, so that he could find any available information on this subject. Although few people in the medical community professed interest in—or awareness of—silicone hazards in the late 1980s, his efforts unearthed a multitude of silicone-related articles dating back to the 1960s. This impressive collection of articles, of which he made copies for me, related many early indications of the perils of silicone. Possibly I knew that another stage of my silicone experiences had begun.

Although I continued to improve, I still had to compensate for a loss of muscular strength which limited physical exertion. So I began talking to Dr. Roach by telephone from my home and I also began speaking with other knowledgeable physicians and researchers. My knowledge of silicone's history started to grow. I learned that silicone had been discovered in the 1930s. However, the substance was not utilized until the 1940s, when Dow Chemical Company and Corning Glass Works, in association with the American military, perfected silicone's industrial use as a lubricant, a sealant and a coolant. In Japan, during the late 1940s, Japanese doctors were among the first to conduct human experiments with a liquid form of silicone injected directly into women's breasts for cosmetic enlargements. This had dire results. The same experimentation in the United States produced a similar negative outcome.[1] Despite this, Dow Corning researchers were undaunted, and began research and development projects in an effort to find other medical applications for silicone. In 1962, they announced the invention of the first silicone breast implant. However, it was McGhan Medical Corporation which first marketed a more flexible, less rubbery implant employing a fluid-gel state of silicone in 1972. By this time, medical research literature had already reported some implant related problems.

The early accounts of routine and continual gel leakage through intact implant shells, which are semi-permeable, were published in the 1970s.[2] Other articles noted the incidence of spontaneous implant ruptures.[3] In studies of implants surgically removed, the most common complications cited were gel loss and capsular contracture, which is the formation of a constricting, fibrous layer around the prosthesis. Problems arising from the contracture, which occurs in forty to seventy percent of all implantations, were reported in the 1970s.[4] This condition often exerts pressure on the implant and increases the leakage of the silicone gel. There were reports that treating the contracture by the application of non-surgical, external compression to break up the fibrous bands sometimes resulted in a rupture of the implant.[5] Since the majority of these research papers and others were published in reconstructive surgery journals, it is possible that many surgeons did not know or consider their significance.

The ability of escaped silicone to travel via the circulatory and lymphatic system, either by gel "bleed" or rupture, was also reported in medical literature twenty years ago.[6] Silicone has been described as having the identical "beaded" appearance that was detected in my own hepatic artery.[7] When I found out these things, I began to comprehend the implications of all I had been experiencing because of my silicone implants.

I learned that silicone has been found in practically every organ and gland of the bodies of those who have had implants, including the spleen, liver, kidneys, ureters, adrenals, uterus, uterine tubes, ovaries, lungs, brain and in inflamed joint lining.[8] This migration results in the development of silicone granulomas, which are non-cancerous lumps, and lymphadenopathy (enlarged and/or diseased lymph nodes). The occurrences of these silicone formations have been reported in medical papers since the 1970s.[9]

Although the chemical industry had reported from the beginning that silicone was harmless, contrary evidence was plentiful in medical literature. It supported the position that silicone is biochemically reactive.[10] My own allergy to silicone verified this position. The immune system can respond to any foreign body. Lymphadenopathy and silicone granulomas are both examples of chronic foreign body reactions; capsular contracture is also a reaction to a foreign substance in the body. The contracture is formed as macrophages, which are white cells that engulf foreign invaders, migrate to the implant and stimulate the collagen deposition.

This condition is an indication that the body recognizes the implant as a foreign object and, in response, tries to reject it by producing tissue to "wall" off the implant from the rest of the body. The severe breast pain I experienced soon after my implantation, I now understood, to be a result of this inflammatory process. I found many other examples of silicone-induced foreign body reaction in the medical literature I read.[11] There are references, from as early as 1974, to histologic changes from silicone concentration in the human breast, hypercalcemia associated with silicone granulomas and numerous accounts of foreign body reaction to silicone gel in lymph nodes throughout the body. This includes lymphadenopathy with a joint inflammation known as synovitis.

Silicone's ability as a foreign invader to induce chronic inflammation is important and often may be a cause of illness. Any implanted foreign material is capable of setting off an immune response. Some will result in a consequent inflammatory illness. According to reports in early medical literature, one radical development that can spring from the sites of embedded medical devices in the body is cancer.[12] The reports of correlations between angiosarcoma and dacron grafts, fibrosarcoma and prosthetic vascular grafts, breast cancer and pacemaker generators are but a few such associations that supply confirming evidence.

At a February 1992 symposium sponsored by the Toxicology Forum in Washington, D.C., Dr. Jerry Rice, National Cancer Institute pathologist and director of the Laboratory of Comparative Carcinogenesis, presented a paper entitled "Solid State Carcinogenesis," which further illustrated the risk of foreign body cancer. He concluded:

> On the basis of forty-six, well-documented cases of
> sarcomas in humans that have been associated with the
> presence of foreign bodies, both metallic and non-metallic,
> it appears that implanted foreign bodies have the capacity to
> induce virtually any form of sarcoma in humans, and that,
> while the risk appears to be very low, it certainly is real.

Dr. Rice's conclusion was not the first of its kind. As early as 1961, one research paper raised the question that silicone implants might be a carcinogenic agent.[13] A succession of published research also linked silicone to cancer. From the late 1970s, medical literature articles described implant-related foreign body sarcoma, silicone lymphadenopathy with attending malignant Lymphoma, neoplasms and carcinomata induced by implant material and malignant Lymphoma with refractive particles present—all of which followed silicone implantation.[14]

# TORN ILLUSIONS

A number of papers reported both malignant Lymphoma and metastatic carcinoma concurring with silicone granulomas.

Despite these reports, during these years physicians were recommending and performing hundreds of thousands of implantations with silicone breast prostheses.

Later, I discovered research that Dow Corning, the largest breast implant manufacturer and silicone supplier, had been testing silicone's carcinogenicity through animal experiments conducted in the late 1960s (Chapters V and VIII). To me, it seemed that industrial investigators failed to publicize their findings for selfish reasons. However, this information was reported for years in many journals. Though the information was available, no one in the medical community warned the public.

Now, women who had silicone implants were becoming increasingly concerned about breast cancer. This concern was well founded. A 1985 medical study which explored the relationship of free silicone to human breast cancer, supports their apprehension.[15] Taking into account the occurrence of gel "bleed" and implant rupture in women, the results were significant.

One study of twelve women with carcinoma of the breast and co-existent silicone mastopathy revealed that nine had received injections of liquid silicone, and three had leaking silicone breast implants. The pathological findings were indicative of an adverse effect from the presence of free silicone within these women's breast tissue, auxiliary lymph nodes and auxiliary fat.

The results of this research did not surprise me, as I had located even earlier evidence of liquid silicone danger. Reports of malignant tumors following breast injections with silicone have been reported in medical literature since the 1960s.[16] There are also published accounts of silicone toxicity and a distribution of silicone in body tissue causing fatalities as a result of this practice. One unfortunate women died ten hours after her breast was injected with silicone.[17] At her autopsy, histologic tissue examination showed the presence of silicone in the woman's lungs, kidneys, liver, brain and blood serum. Her cause of death was reported as "severe acute bilateral pulmonary edema secondary to intravascular silicone injection."

In the early years, the silicone injections used for breast enlargement often included an adulteration of various oils and additives. For a long period, Dow Corning researchers blamed these other substances for the regrettable repercussions of silicone injections. "However," according to one scientist, "even pure medical-grade silicone injected by licensed investigators has provoked toxicity in all degrees. Medical-grade silicone originally was not made for injection, and even it contains impurities."[17] These hazardous injections had never been approved and were eventually banned by the FDA.[18]

In animal studies conducted in 1965 involving primates, injections of pure, unadulterated silicone caused the destruction of the breast anatomies of the animals tested. A 1978 study concluded that silicone gel should not be used in human bodies by "direct instillation" because of the progressive changes noted in subcutaneous sites. Another study in the same year stated that silicone gel must not be "instilled" in humans due to the risks of its phagocytosis (the process by which macrophages engulf foreign substances), and the consequent spread of silicone throughout the body, which caused stimulation of the immune system.

In a court testimony, Mr. Robert Riley, president of Dow Corning Wright, stated that the previously used liquid silicone and the silicone gel contained in breast implants are chemically one and the same.[19]

Since even at these early stages research had already been conducted into silicone gel's perpetual leakage through porous implant shells, as well as the prostheses' high rate of rupture, I think it is unconscionable that Dow Corning and the rest of the implant industry continued to market these implant devices that are only "vehicles" for delivering and distributing free silicone.[20] It seems to me highly unlikely that corporate directors, researchers and scientists did not know that ruinous results, human illnesses and even death could occur.

After all, the first report of many, which related silicone to autoimmune/connective-tissue disease, came from a 1964 publication regarding silicone breast injections.[21] The author of this first research paper invented the term "Human Adjuvant Disease" to describe disorders suspected of being induced by silicone. If silicone, a foreign invader, is introduced into the body, the body can respond with an inflammatory reaction. The production of antibodies is the immune system's normal response to a foreign substance or antigen. An adjuvant is any substance that enhances this immune response. Silicone may be considered such a substance (Chapter VII), hence the name "Human Adjuvant Disease". The result of a persistent inflammatory reaction can be the body's attack of its own tissue, which is autoimmune illness.

At the same time I was discovering these early reports, I learned that Dr. John Heggers of the University of Texas had begun studies in the 1970s which involved the human immune system's ability to produce antibodies in response to silicone. (Dr. Heggers would be contacted by Dr. Finegold to test my own blood serum.) Dr. Heggers made his early research available to officials at Dow Corning in 1978. The company did not pursue this subject.

Nonetheless, independent researchers continued silicone antibody studies. A medical paper, authored by Dr. Heggers and his colleagues, appeared in the 1993 British medical journal *Lancet*, presenting proof of the human production of antibodies to silicone. [22] This was determined by a study of two hydrocephalic children who experienced a severe inflammation from the implanted silicone tubing that assisted in the treatment of their birth defects. Dr. Heggers found that antibodies were attaching to the silicone tubing inside of these children. The serum from five other children with tube implants who did not experience reactions and the serum of nine healthy adults exhibited no similar antibody binding.

Medical researchers have also theorized for some time that silicone may produce autoimmune illness by converting itself into silica, a substance long evidenced to have a profound effect on the human immune system. The inhalation of silica often results in a lung disease, silicosis, found in coal miners due to their exposure to silica. This serious condition is chronic, progressive and usually fatal. Silica, a cytotoxic substance with the ability to kill cells, can cause lung cancer as well. Research of the cytotoxic action of silica was published in 1963. [23] In a current medical paper entitled "Autoimmunity and

Nervous System Dysfunction Associated with Silicone Breast Implants," Dr. Bernard Patten of Baylor College of Medicine in Houston discussed the silica/silicone connection:

> It has become clear that silicone is not at all biologically nor chemically inactive.... It has been demonstrated that silicone and silica are cytotoxic and immunostimulatory agents.... Both silicone and silica elicit a cellular immune and humoral response, acting as hapten-like incomplete antigens. Macrophages might produce silica from phagocytized silicone through an NADP pathway, an important concept for silica itself is mutagenic. Systemic scleroderma and systemic lupus have been reported in individuals with occupational silicone exposure.[24]

Not long ago, I was jarred by the discovery that the potentially deadly silica is—and has been since the device's inception—included in both silicone gel and in all implant shells (Chapter VI).[25]

The first reports that linked silicone implantation to the same inflammatory immune diseases associated previously with silicone breast injections were published in medical literature as early as 1982. [26] The papers reported on the development of autoimmune phenomenon and connective-tissue disease following breast implantation with classic examples of scleroderma, systemic sclerosis, lupus erythematosus, rheumatoid arthritis, Hashimoto's thyroiditis and both Raynaud's as well as Sjogren's syndromes.

I continued my detective work.

One of the articles I read was especially horrifying for me. In published studies of systemic sclerosis, which had developed in four women after their silicone implantation, all exhibited evidence of silicone leakage.[27] Silicone with resulting chronic inflammation had been found in tissue distant from the implant. The authors were of the opinion that this evidence of silicone's propensity for migration, as well as its capacity to elicit inflammatory responses, implicated silicone in the development of these women's diseases. Other non-diagnostic examples of systemic illness relating to silicone implants were also cited. One case involved a woman who almost died from kidney failure before the removal of her prostheses.[28] A particularly disturbing aspect of the reported implant-associated illnesses was what researchers call the "latency period," a time during which symptoms might lay dormant and not materialize until six to fifteen years or longer after implantation. Reading it, I had to admit to myself I might never be free.

The implant's envelope (or shell), which contains the interior fill of silicone gel or saline, was identified in some medical literature as another source of concern.[29] Silicone particles reportedly shed from the outer shells and polyurethane-coated envelopes were found to be even more problematic. Fragments of polyurethane have even been detected embedded in some patients' chest walls. In one instance, the polyurethane foam completely separated itself from the implant shell, due to the growth of fibrous tissue. Tissue reactions to the polyurethane-coated implants were noted, as was the dissolution of the polyurethane foam within the body. (Polyurethane-coated implants are discussed in Chapters V and VIII.)

Although the numerous reports in medical literature over the last thirty years highlight silicone's relationship to human illness and provide ample forewarning, these red flags were ignored. As many looked the other way, an estimated 130,000 American women, and many thousands more in other countries, were implanted yearly with silicone breast prostheses.[30] Silicone's potential for producing illness, combined with the large number of implantations, set the stage for a crisis of vast proportion and repercussion.

In the late 1980s, there was growing media coverage of the cases of reported illness. Many women were as astonished as I was upon finding out about not only silicone breast implants' propensity for causing medical problems, but also the scope and magnitude of these problems. They, too, slowly became aware of having been subjected to unknown risks from a product they believed safe. However, the extent of the implant recipients' exposure still was not realized until several years later.

At this point, some of those who had already sustained implant-related injuries sought legal representation, armed with the knowledge that they were not isolated cases. Lawyers acquired an interest in product liability litigation. At the time, awareness was growing.

I had just bought a townhouse in the Las Olas area of Fort Lauderdale and had begun to achieve some semblance of a normal life for my children and myself. Throughout the earlier years of my convalescence, I had continued to lease different apartments while awaiting the return of my physical strength. When Teresa married and moved back to the Virgin Islands in 1988, I finally found and bought a home because I felt relatively able, with the help of my children, to manage on my own. Nevertheless, I was not yet strong, nor well enough for employment.

Although my divorce settlement was more than adequate, I had incurred significant financial losses during my years of illness because of the continuous medical bills and the loss of income.

The knowledge that I was not alone led me to think of initiating my own legal action. I talked to Dr. Roach, who also suggested that I consider legal counseling, as would many silicone victims. A short while later I contacted my attorney, Bruno Di Guilian. He recommended that I talk to product liability lawyers and arranged a consultation. I also consulted with the law firm of Papy, Weissenborn and Papy. I felt they were the right ones for the case.

James McMaster, an enterprising attorney associated with that firm, decided to collect my tissue samples from my 1985 operations, which were stored in hospital pathology banks. Then he submitted the specimens for pathology examination. Silicone was found in my breast tissue samples; evidence of silicone gel loss through the bleed process.

During this same period, Dr. Finegold sent a sample of my blood serum to Dr. Heggers, a researcher in Texas. Heggers' testing determined the presence of silicone antibodies in these blood samples. Later, when I spoke to Dr. Heggers concerning my test results, I asked, "Do you know of other cases similar to mine?"

He said "I hear from different women in many parts of the United States, who each tell me a comparable 'horror story.'"

A shiver ran down my spine as I realized the magnitude of silicone's destructiveness. However, I had not yet witnessed or felt its

# TORN ILLUSIONS

total impact, even upon my own life. Although my medical problems were slowly resolving, a legal nightmare which lasted many more years was beginning.

In June of 1989, shortly after Dr. Finegold confirmed that my illness and the ensuing medical problems were a result of my silicone implantation, James McMaster filed my product liability action against Dow Corning and Heyer-Schulte. I had never before been involved in a litigation. Therefore, due to my naivete and my heart-felt belief that I had justifiable cause for legal action, I expected the manufacturers to accept responsibility for both their product and my injuries.

On the contrary, the filing of my lawsuit began a long, bitter legal entanglement with manufacturers and their lawyers. As time went on I wondered how the emotional torment on women like me, who were already physically injured, could be justified. If this was an attempt to discourage the growing numbers of lawsuits brought by those of us harmed by silicone, it failed. The legal problems of those who had manufactured silicone devices worsened. Both the victims and the general public stood alerted and were prepared to fight.

Women who had silicone implants and were in need of medical and legal assistance began to organize. The formation of Command Trust Network (CTN), a support organization for silicone illness, opened up a lifeline of communication for injured women in the United States (Appendix). They were now able to contact one another and, once in touch, were able to share information and resources. In addition, local support groups formed in United States' cities and in many other countries support groups also sprang up. These afforded comfort to the growing numbers of those afflicted throughout the world.

# 5

# INVESTIGATIONS BEGIN

In February of 1989, Dr. Finegold received the Food and Drug Administration's first public acknowledgment that illness and injury can occur in association with silicone breast implantation. The alert, in the form of a letter mailed by the agency to physicians, arrived with an enclosed adverse reaction form.[1] Meanwhile, I had already uncovered evidence of the implant's potential for harm when Dr. Finegold returned the FDA form with a report of my own silicone allergy and implant-related toxic illness.

My attention then shifted to the FDA, a government bureau instituted for the public's protection. I was greatly interested in the role played by the agency in allowing silicone prostheses to be marketed without precautions or warnings. The evidence I had seen made me feel sure that the prostheses had never been proven safe, and I saw no proof that the regulatory agency had investigated their safety, despite several decades of breast implant use. As I continued searching medical journals and the FDA's past announcements involving silicone, I learned that this oversight began with the agency's classification of medical devices. My feelings about the FDA's poor performance in the silicone drama were becoming stronger.

Medical devices were not regulated by the FDA until 1976. At that time, a new congressional law gave the agency the power to do so. The Medical Device Act of 1976 mandated that all medical devices be classified in one of three required categories: Category I-labeling; Category II-performance; and Category III-pre-market approval. While trying to determine the route of the silicone implant through the FDA's safety net of classification, I spoke to Kathleen Anneken, founder of the national support group, Command Trust Network (CTN). Kathleen directed me to Jerry Kuester, Medical Devices Researcher at the Public Citizens Health Research Group (PCHRG), an organization committed to serving the public while watching over both industry and government. Mr. Kuester helpfully supplied me with much information about the FDA's regulation of medical devices.

While studying all the information I could find I learned that the initial Panel on Review of General and Plastic Devices met in 1974 in preparation for the enactment of new legislation. Due to the fact that silicone implants had been available for fifteen years, the panel originally recommended placing the devices in Category II (exempt from new product testing). Over the next few years, however, reports of implant rupture, leakage, associated information and hardening of the breasts increased at a steady pace, and many on the FDA staff sought the devices' reclassification to Category III, a status requiring product safety data from the manufacturers in order to secure the necessary pre-market approval (PMA) of the prostheses.

While wading through FDA papers and other information, I read transcripts about several General and Plastic Surgery Device Classification Panel Reviews, held in 1978, to address the growing concerns over breast implant safety.[2] At this early date, the FDA had heard, but did not react to, the first sounding of an alarm. In March of the same year, Dr. Henry Jenny, inventor of the saline implant currently in use, presented the review panel with strong evidence of the gel's leakage through the porous implant shells. Showing slides of silicone droplets inside small capillaries, he demonstrated silicone's ability to travel via the bloodstream. Dr. Jenny also discussed the long-range hazards of silicone inflammation and cancer, further predicting that "within fifteen years" symptoms of illness would surface in silicone-implanted women.[3]

At a July General and Plastic Surgery Section, Surgical, and Rehabilitation Device Panel Review, Dr. J.L. Abraham, a pathologist at the University of Chicago, furnished evidence of silicone's presence in tissue distant from an intact gel-filled implant. He warned that metabolic and other effects of prolonged exposure to silicone when inside the body were unknown. During the same July meeting, Dr. R. LeVier, technical director of Dow Corning's Health Care Business, reviewed the company's toxicology data. Utilizing the manufacturer's own studies, the panel reported on not only the gel-bleed of the Dow Corning implant, but also the development of inflammatory responses to free silicone.

In spite of convincing testimony and evidence warning of possible problems from silicone implants brought forth during preliminary reviews, an October 18, 1979 FDA Panel Review upheld their standing recommendations. Thus, the devices retained their Category II classification. Without the product safety provisions of a higher Category III, the silicone implant continued to be marketed and widely used over another decade. The necessity for an extended, comprehensive study concerning the consequence of implant use was clearly evident at this time, yet studies were not—nor would they be—conducted.

It seemed obvious to me that the industry vehemently opposed the reclassification of silicone implants, which would require proving the devices safe. As I digested all the material I'd read, I thought it highly improbable that the manufacturers would enter into such fierce combat to prevent the disclosure of safety data if their product could, indeed, be proven a safe one. I felt it was an early indication that such safety information did not exist. If the conclusion of unproven safety had been reached at the beginning of medical device regulation, with subsequent implant reclassification, it is not likely that I would have decided to become an implant recipient and so I would not have then been an eventual silicone victim. While reflecting on this, I realized that by the year of my implantation, the devices had gained in popularity and had become a thriving business for both industry and plastic surgeons. Many resisted silicone implant reclassification as well as FDA interference.

The war between those who wanted silicone implants to be reclassified and those who didn't continued. Within two years, the FDA received thousands of implant-related complaints and data. These reports added evidence to the theory that increasingly linked systemic and autoimmune illnesses to silicone implantation. However, once again, some in the agency proposed reclassification.

During the period before the proposal, an announcement in the Federal Register listed the reasons for the projected move to Category III as the migration of gel "with or without rupture," the "contraction of the fibrous capsule" around the implant and the "possible long-term toxic effects."[4]

It was during the time that the FDA's projected reclassification was first announced that I experienced "toxic effects." My physicians were not yet aware or informed of any vulnerability to illness arising from a woman's implantation with these popular devices. I believe that a major reason for the difficulty and delay in accurately diagnosing my illness—as the silicone bled, traveled, and played havoc throughout my entire system—was the lack of published information. It is very difficult to accept the fact that the FDA possessed it and did nothing. A great deal of my suffering could have been relieved if the implants were removed three years earlier. This would have been possible had the information been disseminated among the medical community. A considerable number of other implant recipients were equally affected by the agency's muteness.

Despite the attempt that year to change the category in which the FDA had put silicone, silicone implant problems remained shrouded in obscurity.

Many physicians and patients were kept in the dark, while breast enlargement operations, being conducted on millions of unsuspecting women, moved forward uninterrupted. Not until June 24, 1988, six years after the proposal was introduced, did the FDA complete the reclassification of the silicone implants to Category III and finally give full legal notice to the industry that the submission of safety data—a requirement of this classification—would be enforced.

The law provided a thirty month grace period for manufacturers to comply with the pre-market approval (PMA) regulations, which caused another dangerous delay. The Federal Register notice of June 24, 1988, stated:

> FDA has examined recent scientific data concerning silicone
> implants and the migration of silicone in the body that
> support the agency's proposed classification. Some of these
> data reveal the occurrence of allergic reactions, silicone
> lymphadenoma, morbidity due to silicone and silicone
> migration.[5]

By that year, it is undeniable that many cases of serious illness were reported among women with implants. These findings were not made public, nor did the FDA enforce the manufacturers' mandatory notification of known implant risks. Additionally, the agency did not initiate an implant patient registry, although such a program was recommended as a necessity in the report as well as the follow-up of implant-related injuries.

Another concern, which was not included in the FDA's June announcement but was later mentioned in the agency's November "Talk Paper," related to silicone/fetal toxicity. The paper, which was not distributed outside of the agency, disclosed that some reports had indicated that "small quantities of gel have been shown to migrate throughout the body, and this has raised questions about possible effects on the immune system and the fetus."[6] (Silicone implant-related fetal risk and female reproductive system involvement are discussed in Chapter VIII.)

Although I lost my ovaries to silicone while young, fortunately, I had already conceived two children. Many young women may not be as fortunate. Any woman with implants also runs the risk of passing on implant-associated hazards to their unborn children.

In November, the FDA convened another panel review about the specifications of the PMA data to be submitted by the manufacturers.[7] During the proceedings, Dow Corning requested that the company's biosafety research be held in strict confidence, referring to a 1985 through 1987 laboratory study using rats. In accordance with this request, the FDA did not release this information, although these particular animal studies revealed the silicone implant could be carcinogenic (Chapter VIII).

Attorney Dan Bolton of California also attended the 1988 panel review. Mr. Bolton had represented the plaintiff in an implant litigation in the case of Stern vs. Dow Corning four years earlier. At the close of this trial, the jury imposed a $1.5 million punitive damage award against Dow Corning. Afterward, all accusatory corporate documents entered in court during that trial were sealed; lawyers for Dow Corning asked for a protective order preventing their future disclosure (Chapter IX). As a result, court records were sealed by protective ordersin twenty cases.

Regarding the sealed trial documents, Mr. Bolton testified:

> I can tell you, however, that the jury saw many of these
> documents and determined that DOW had committed
> fraud, misled the public, and disregarded the safety of
> women in marketing silicone breast implants. The judge in
> the Stern case described Dow's conduct as, quote,'highly
> reprehensible.'[8]

I was involved in my own litigation when I came across information pertaining to the Stern trial against Dow Corning and its outcome. Reading all the data I wondered what other reason than self-interest could account for Dow's position on not divulging information to the public. After Dow Corning requested that the company's cancer data be suppressed (as other data had been) due to a fear of public furor, the agency conformed, citing as a reason "corporate competition."

At this time, the FDA had not obtained proof of silicone implant safety, yet the agency did have current evidence of implant risks. Nevertheless, it was not until May 17, 1990, that the Federal Register published the long-awaited proposal requiring the filing of PMA applications. These were intended to be submitted to the agency by August 15, 1990, with all petitions for a change of classification based on "new information" due by June 1, 1990. Written comments of "interested persons" were to be presented by July 16, 1990. The FDA approved and granted filing extensions.

In late 1990, Representative Ted Weiss, Chairman of the House Subcommittee on Human Resources and Intergovernmental Relations, queried the FDA as to why there was a delay in completing the silicone implant's pre-market approval. A Congressional hearing followed, during which physicians gave testimony concerning the occurrence of breast implant-associated illness. Around the time of the publicized hearings, Connie Chung put together a television segment, as did *60 Minutes*, addressing implant safety concerns, which were by then a national issue. After the producer of the *Connie Chung Show* learned of my own silicone illness through support group contacts, she asked for my participation in a summer taping for the upcoming program. Unfortunately, I was already scheduled to give dispositions in my product liability case and so was unable to accept the invitation.

Prior to the hearings on my case, I submitted a summary of my silicone-related medical documentation to Paul Tilton of the FDA. Later, Jerry Kuester of the Public Citizen Health Research Group (PGHRG), routed the summary directly to Commissioner Kessler. Many were questioning whether or not agency officials correctly assimilated the illness data when reported. In addition, the Congressional Subcommittee, which Representative Weiss chaired, had begun looking into the FDA's regulation of breast implants.

As a result of the heightened media attention, public pressure began to grow. An FDA sponsored conference, convened in February of 1991, included discussions of silicone-immune toxicity and autoimmune illness, which further illuminated the lack of implant safety data. Two months later, the agency issued a final rule and a request for safety data to be submitted within ninety days. Upon finishing an evaluation of the material, the FDA made a formal ruling on January 6, 1992.[9]

Silicone implant manufacturers affected by the PMA requirements were Dow Corning, McGhan, Mentor, Baxter Healthcare, Bioplasty, Surgitex, Cox-Uphoft and Ponex. Although Dow Corning drew the most publicity and was the company the public most focused upon because of the release of the company's damaging animal studies and corporate memorandums, analogous testing was standard procedure among many implant manufacturers. Five salesmen and scientists had originally left Dow Corning, taking with them their acquired knowledge of silicone implant manufacturing. After contributing their data and skills to Heyer-Schulte, in 1974 the group opened McGhan Medical Corporation. The resulting corporate mergers and buyouts form most of today's implant industry.

Despite the PMA ruling, not all implant manufacturers complied with the data requirements. However, when the FDA scientists studied the submissions of four companies that did provide the information, they concluded that the evidence was not sufficient to establish the devices' safety. The FDA next scheduled a November convening of a twenty-two member advisory panel to review the increasingly questionable safety status of silicone-gel implants.

By the fall of 1991, as the review approached, my recovery had begun to stabilize. My day-to-day living circumstances improved as my health problems lessened. I found I had a greater degree of energy and I soon became more involved in the problems of other implant patients, many of whom were just beginning to experience implant-related illnesses or were still recovering from having their implants removed. One group in which I participated was a silicone support group, founded by Teri Davis and Nina Flinn. The organization offered counseling for implant patients, but both women felt overexerted from the time and effort that the support work demanded. Often ill herself, and unable to speak to the many women who contacted her daily, Teri frequently asked me to take some of her calls and perform this service.

Most of the women to whom I spoke knew very little about the emerging research on silicone implantation. A large number had just recently had silicone implants and were uninformed of any associated risks. Although it was too late to retrieve my own stolen past, I was particularly concerned that others should not be similarly robbed. It was my belief, from first hand experience in my own litigation, that the manufacturers wouldn't accept responsibilities to these victimized women and would keep their products on the market while more unaware women were harmed.

Meanwhile, the FDA scientists had recently determined the implant's safety to be unproven, and many women were already experiencing the consequences of having implants in their bodies. Therefore, I intently watched the proceedings of their important November review, for both personal and impersonal reasons, wary of both the industry's vested interests in silicone and the FDA's policy making.

As it turned out, the advisory members of the FDA, during the meeting, agreed with the agency's scientists that the manufacturers' data was insufficient, failing to support product safety.[10] The panel, nonetheless, recommended the continued availability of the devices due to a public health care need for silicone implants.

However, they added the restrictions that an informed consent and patient registry be provided. In the meantime, the manufacturers would collect additional safety information over a three-year period.

The claim that American women had a health care need for silicone implants provided the manufacturers with more time. Due to a "loophole" in the 1976 Medical Device Act, the law permits a medical product to remain on the market even if it fails to be proven safe, as long as, collaterally, a valid health care need for the product can be established. The FDA format of the November panel review seemed to me to devote a disproportionate amount of time toward authenticating the health need of American women for silicone implants. They cited implants' use by cancer patients in reconstructive surgery as one example.

Forced to justify the eighty-five percent of breast augmentations which are performed for cosmetic improvement, the panel referred to the psychological need for women to feel more attractive.[11] One panelist felt that the prostheses were a necessity for many women who believe they function in society as "beauty objects." I could not help being resentful and wondering just who they thought had sold women this definition of themselves. Also objecting to this suggestion, Dr. Sidney Wolfe, director of the Public Citizen

Health Research Group (PCHRG), said that "it is impossible to believe that the FDA would consider such sexist, outlandish reasoning as constituting a public health need."[12]

The FDA advisory panel forum evoked much criticism. Limited to a review of the manufacturers' inadequate proof of safety for silicone devices, the review assembly did not include or accept proof of harmfulness in the discussions. Dr. Wolfe was one protestor who wrote to Dr. David Kessler, the recently appointed FDA Commissioner. Dr. Wolfe's letter of remonstration stated that the agency "misled" the panel in understating the undisclosed risks.

Several panel members also wrote to Commissioner Kessler complaining of the FDA's obvious influence on the panel's "decision-making process."[13] A letter from Dr. Marc Lappé of the University of Illinois College of Medicine in Chicago, stated:

> I am writing to comment critically about the process used and conclusions reached by the Panel on Silicone Breast Implants that met earlier this month. . . . The decision to vote on public health need was brought out in the last fifteen minutes before we convened November 14, by panelists who believed that their conditional vote the previous day would be recorded as a blanket denial of marketing.[14]

Vivian Snyder, the panel's consumer representative, expressed the following misgivings:

> I am especially concerned about some aspects of the process which I experienced. As an outsider to the FDA it seemed, at times, that the ways in which procedural issues were communicated to the panel [the FDA] might have been subtly guiding us to the conclusion that silicone implants were indeed a public health issue.[14]

Another controversial point related to the manufacturers' preselection of the experts who testified before the advisory panel. Panel member Dr. Norman Anderson, Johns Hopkins School of Medicine in Baltimore, wrote:

> By designating an advisory panel of 11 voting members where only 4 had any semblance of familiarity with breast

implants, the FDA created a body of novices susceptible to one-sided testimony of experts selected by the manufacturers. . . . In such a tilted playing field, the opinions of psychologists and psychiatrists, who have studied only the happier outcomes of breast implant usage, easily carried the day for the manufacturers, while the testimony of ten women clearly injured by failed implant surgery was dismissed as anecdotal irrelevance.[14]

Dr. Anderson, who had stated his concerns over implant safety and had served on the FDA advisory panel from 1982, would, in the February 1992 panel review, lose his status as a voting member. However, he did continue to serve on the advisory panel in a nonvoting capacity.

Many people raised objections regarding the FDA dealings with the manufacturers on the breast implant issue. According to the Human Resources and Intergovernmental Relations Subcommittee, which investigated the FDA's management of the silicone implant controversy, staff members and scientists at the agency had been reporting implant problems for fifteen years.[15] Some said concerns and recommendations were ignored, and even obstructed, by high-ranking senior officials. This became a matter of much speculation.

By the end of 1991, I had gathered additional pertinent information in support of the subcommittee's findings. Some of the things I found out were that, as far back as 1965, the FDA declared silicone injections illegal unless a physician had a permit to conduct human experiments.[16] By 1978, the agency had been alerted to incidence of implant rupture and gel leakage, as well as resulting silicone inflammation. Occurrences of silicone-associated illness with immune system involvement were repeatedly reported to the agency. In 1982, the FDA concluded that "the silicone implant presents a potentially unreasonable risk of injury," yet the devices remained unsupervised and readily available for another ten years.[17] While the FDA complied with the manufacturers' requests, women were left unprotected and at the mercy of manufacturers who completely "disregarded," as one jury concluded, their health and welfare.

In 1988, the FDA received more bad news about silicone. In that year they were given information that lymphoma, a malignant tumor of the lymphatic system, occurred in eighty percent (an audit later determined it to be one hundred percent) of the test animals exposed to silicone gel. The two year (1985-1987) Dow Corning study, which the company's lawyers asked the FDA not to release, further determined silicone's inducement of fibrosarcoma (an extremely lethal soft tissue malignancy) in twenty-three percent of the silicone-implanted laboratory animals.

Eighty-five percent of these animals eventually died of their malignancies.[18] A 1988 FDA memorandum in summary of the Dow Corning cancer research data stated: "Silicone can cause cancer in rats; there is no direct proof silicone causes cancer in humans; however, there is considerable reason to suspect that silicone can do so."[19] Although the agency claimed they did not have conclusive proof of a silicone/cancer relationship in human beings, they had convincing reports of its occurrence.

A May 1990 Federal Register publication stated:

> Some clinicians have reported malignant Lymphoma and metastatic carcinoma concurrently with silicone granulomas. . . . Carcinogenicity has been a widely discussed topic related to the injection of silicone fluid in augmentation mammaplasty since the early 1950s. . . .the potential for developing cancer as a long-term complication related to silicone migration remains a potential risk associated with the implants.[20]

This information was not presented to the November 1991 advisory panel, whose decision would affect the lives of many innocent women. Neither did the FDA alert these women to the risk of cancer.

In 1988, Dr. Sidney Wolfe had written FDA Commissioner Young about the agency's own evidence of silicone's cancer-causing potential and implored the commissioner "to halt immediately the use of silicone gel materials for implantation in the human body." The Public Citizen Health Research Group, founded by Ralph Nader and Dr. Wolfe, subsequently petitioned to have the implants banned.

# TORN ILLUSIONS

During that same year, Dr. M. L. Luu, a conscientious FDA scientist involved in the agency's study of silicone implants, made two recommendations:

> That a medical alert be issued to warn the public of the
> possibility of malignancy development in humans
> following long-term implant of silicone breast prostheses
> and that mandatory leaflet information regarding adverse
> reactions and risk of silicone prostheses given to past,
> present and future patients.[21]

The FDA did not enact these recommendations, but instead, removed Dr. Luu and Dr. N. Mishra, another critic within the FDA, from their work in the silicone implant field. The members of a November 1988 advisory panel considered, as well, recommendations similar to those of Dr. Luu and Dr. Mishra that both a warning of the cancer risk be issued to women with silicone implants and appropriate changes be made in the manufacturers' package insert sent to physicians and patients. These recommendations were not implemented either. The same panel recognized the need for silicone/fetotoxicity data, which the FDA had never required, nor did they initiate a research program in this area.[22]

Furthermore, women were not told of the slightest possibility of fetal risk, yet the agency had received reports of many risks; to me their failure to issue a public warning on their part is deplorable and truly inexcusable. It appears that scientific, medical and laboratory data were shuffled about, then not released by our "protective" federal agency. However, it is indisputable that laboratory findings hold a great deal of relevancy for human application.

The drug, Diethylstilbestrol (DES), is one ominous example of a dangerous substance that was administered to women, despite strong evidence of its harmful effects. Studies showed that DES could induce cancer in test animals, yet it was administered to prevent miscarriage in humans.[23] This treatment resulted in the development of breast cancer in many of the mothers and the development of cancer of the reproductive organs in many of their daughters years later.[24]

Like the mothers who took DES, the majority of women with breast implants are unaware of their own exposure to unacceptable risks, the magnitude of which the FDA has never publicly acknowledged or disclosed.

At the core of this problem is the FDA's decision to allow manufacturers confidentiality, rather than to alert the public. Because of this decision, some have taken legal action against the FDA. In 1989, the Public Citizens Health Research Group sued the agency in an attempt to make public the thousands of pages of Dow Corning animal studies and documents that were withheld by the agency. Washington Federal Judge Stanley Sporkin, also vexed by the FDA's refusal to relinquish the Dow Corning cancer studies, signed a court order for their release. He stated, reproaching the FDA, "An agency cannot pretend that it has not seen information, especially information relating to a public danger."[25] Dow Corning intervened as codefendant with the FDA, and appeals shortly followed.

When, in March of 1991, a New York jury found the polyurethane-coated silicone implant to have caused a woman's breast cancer, the FDA was again under fire. The trial ended with an award of $4.45 million against Natural Y Surgical Specialties of Los Angeles.[26] One month later, Surgitek (a subsidiary of Bristol-Myers Squibb and a large manufacturer distributing the polyurethane-coated implants) removed the devices from the market due to polyurethane's breakdown to TDA (2-toulene diamine), which was shown to produce liver cancer in research animals. [27]

The FDA took the position that the risk associated with TDA was "very small" and blamed the media for creating "an unnecessary climate of fear." In rebuttal, Representative Ted Weiss charged the FDA with downgrading the degree of TDA risk, charging that the agency's reassurances did "not accurately reflect the conclusions of FDA's own scientists." In a letter to Commissioner Kessler citing the internal documents of the FDA scientists, Representative Weiss wrote: "In fact, the cancer risks ... may be one hundred times the level reported by FDA and by Surgitek, the manufacturer."[28]

Representative Weiss also chastised the agency for not disclosing the risk of possible birth defects, which the FDA had listed

# TORN ILLUSIONS

as the very reason for the ban of TDA's use in hair dyes in the 1970s. [29] He concluded that "some at FDA became more concerned with the reputation of the manufacturer than informing the public." The FDA, the National Toxicology Program and the International Agency for Research on Cancer have "categorized" TDA as a "potential human carcinogen."[30] Approximately 200,000 to 400,000 women have been implanted with this particular silicone implant.[31]

To this day, the FDA does not conduct its own safety testing, but instead relies exclusively on the data supplied by outsiders, much of whose research is funded by the manufacturers themselves. Yet, the PCHRG has already reported violations by thirty-five medical device companies in FDA notifications of adverse reactions.

In routine FDA inspections from 1985 through 1988, the FDA discovered at least seven deaths, 109 serious injuries, 265 malfunctions and seventy-five malfunctions with unspecified serious injury.[32] All went unreported by the manufacturers of the devices.

In addition, in recent years several major drug companies have pleaded guilty to criminal charges filed in conjunction with withholding data from the FDA. As a result of some drug manufacturers having denied the agency this information, possibly potential lethal drugs, which were later banned, gained FDA approval. Some generic drug companies are currently under investigation.[33]

In a November 1991, article about a California case involving Dow Corning, a *Business Week* magazine article stated that "In a way, an entire industry will now be on trial."[34] As a matter of fact, it was. The jury in the highly publicized case ruled that Dow Corning's own research showed that silicone implants presented risks, but that it failed to warn doctors or patients and, thereby, committed fraud and malice. An $840,000 compensatory award and a $6.5 million punitive damage award were subsequently imposed against the corporation. On December 30, 1991, Dan Bolton, the plaintiff's attorney in Hopkins vs. Dow Corning, wrote to FDA Commissioner Kessler informing him of the court-entered documents and testimony.

Seth Rosenfeld, an investigative reporter for *The San Francisco Examiner,* came into possession of the Dow Corning documents. When the FDA refused to accept the papers, Mr. Rosenfeld presented the information to FDA panel member Dr. Norman Anderson. According to the *California Lawyer*, Dr. Anderson was infuriated by the contents of the evidence, and he immediately contacted Commissioner Kessler.[35] Due to these combined efforts, the FDA received many new documents and animal studies that Dow Corning had not previously disclosed to the agency.

On January 6, 1992, Commissioner Kessler announced the beginning of a forty-five day moratorium on the use of silicone breast implants. "Rather than dispelling doubts," he said, "the new information has increased our concerns about the safety of these devices." Commissioner Kessler stated that another advisory committee would be convened in order to review the newly acquired information. Then he asked the advisory committee to reassess its earlier recommendations.

Afterward, Commissioner Kessler ordered Dow Corning to immediately produce all animal studies and internal corporate memorandums. Within hours of the public release of the company's documents on January 11, 1992, Dow Corning replaced some of its top executives. It was rumored some were implicated in the repression of documentation concerning silicone-associated risks. Keith R. McKennon, a long-term board member, was appointed both CEO and Chairman. A week later, Dow Corning stopped the factory production of silicone breast implants.

By this time, plastic surgeons had actively entered the fray. As of 1992, in America alone, women had spent an estimated $4.5 million yearly for silicone breast implant surgery, the second most frequently performed form of cosmetic surgery.[36] As a result of the great deal of money involved, it was rumored that self-interests clouded the judgment of many surgeons, and rationalization was widespread. Plastic surgeons, however, were not swayed by the self-interest of income alone. Implant litigation placed many in legal jeopardy. Wedged between the patient and the manufacturers, they were often included in lawsuits. An FDA ban of the devices they had routinely implanted in thousands of patients would increase their legal vulnerability.

# TORN ILLUSIONS

In response to increasing media attention on silicone implants, the American Society of Plastic and Reconstructive Surgeons (ASPRS) funded a four million dollars campaign to counter adverse implant publicity. These funds launched an advertising and correspondence effort that promptly delivered 20,000 letters to the FDA and Congress. The organization called for the resignation of Commissioner Kessler. The ASPRS further paid the expenses of 400 women to travel to Washington, where they were to lobby Congress as examples of happy implant patients. The society also contributed $62,450 to what was called sixty-one "key" senators and congressmen during 1991-1992.[37]

However, while the surgeons' society fought to preserve the silicone-gel implant, the FDA's toll-free "hotline" fielded thousands of calls from women with implants who were either injured or who had become alarmed.

Much was at stake, and the FDA scheduled another Advisory Panel to convene on February 18, 1992. The future of the silicone breast implant was to be decided. At the meeting, panel members reviewed the Dow Corning internal corporate documents which were presently in their possession. Charges of countless transgressions were be leveled at the corporation. The embarrassment and legal ramifications which would arise from the public airing of dirty corporate laundry evidently effected Dow. The company issued a press statement in which women were advised to have an implant removed in the event of a rupture, and to have as much loose gel as possible scraped from the chest. The company stated that, if the gel could not be removed once outside the shell, it might become "runny" and move to other parts of the body. Dow Corning further stated that, as a result of the gel's migration from the implant site, "the potential exists for medical complications."[38]

Tragically, this acknowledgment from one manufacturer came far too late for me and millions of other women who had already been exposed to silicone. I thought angrily and sadly of the thousands who had been injured and irreparably damaged, and the many lives which have been destroyed or lost.

# TORN ILLUSIONS

When manufacturing representatives and plastic surgeons could no longer refute the strong evidence of the dangers of silicone, many resorted to defining those afflicted as being a "small number." By discounting the victims' numbers, they deemed the issue inconsequential. However, based on a *New York Times* article, three hundred and fifty six women are implanted daily, resulting in approximately one to two million women in the United States alone with silicone breast implants and millions more worldwide.[39] If, as some theorize, only one percent of those women are susceptible to silicone-related illness, the total would now be over 74,333 women in the United States and an even greater number in other countries, such as England, France and Japan.

Many researchers and physicians believe, as I do, that the actual total will be much higher. In fact, implant-related injuries and illnesses (including those resulting in death) in the reports of the manufacturers alone, have already tripled this estimate (Chapter VI). Also, these current figures do not encompass the large number of women in whom latent cancer and autoimmune disease has just begun to occur or will appear later.

In the future, it is predicted that a minimum of ten to fourteen percent—or well over 200,000 women—will be affected.

I often wonder how the manufacturers and surgeons would explain or contend with what they call a "minimum" risk if one person in this, as they have classified it, "small" group of women happened to be one of their own wives, daughters or loved ones.

# 6

## EVIDENCE BECOMES AVAILABLE

My product liability case was on the court docket, and depositions were continuing. Dr. Shanklin had already reported the depressing news that there was silicone in my breast tissue; McAllister, my attorney, decided to have the ovarian pathology tissue from my 1987 surgery tested for the same possibility.

Immersed, as I was, in the anxiety-provoking depositions for my lawsuit against Dow Corning, I pushed my anxious thoughts about the results of the new tests to the back of my mind. Once in a while I called McAllister to ask about them, but he always said, "No news is good news. Let's not worry about the results 'till they're in."

I followed his advice, but I vaguely noted that the test results seemed to be taking a very long time. Nevertheless, I had almost managed to forget this possible added complication when late one evening in the spring, the day before the plastic surgeon who had inserted my implants was due to give his depositions, McAllister telephoned me.

"Pam, I need to see you right away. Can you come down to my office first thing tomorrow morning?"

His grim voice unnerved me. Taking a deep breath, I replied, "Of course. What's up?"

McAllister was uncharacteristically brusque. "I'd rather not talk about it on the phone. I'll see you in the morning," he said and hung up.

The rest of the night inched by. Tossing and turning in my bed, I agonized about what had gone wrong this time.

Early the next morning, I got up, quickly dressed and hurried to his office without even stopping for breakfast. Once there, I parked my car and went right in. Recognizing me, his secretary quickly ushered me from the reception room to McAllister's office.

McAllister, who was seated at his large mahogany desk, rose and strode towards me, some papers in his hand. Without a word he handed them to me. I looked down. It was the report on the ovarian tissue.

Sinking into the nearest chair I read the shocking news that silicone had also invaded my ovaries. McAllister stood nearby watching me.

Lifting my head, I looked into his eyes. "It's one blow after another," I said wearily.

McAllister sighed. "You're very brave, Pam. I don't know how you've held up so well. If it was me, I'd have broken long...."

"So well?" I blurted out, while shaking my head. "I don't think I'm standing up very well right now. I'm trembling so much I can't even read this paper. I'm losing more and more weight, and, except for my children, I have no life. What is 'well?'"

" 'Well' is not accepting defeat. You're a fighter, Pamela, and no matter how tough the battle is, you hang in there."

"I have no choice," I replied, giving a small laugh. "The alternative is even worse."

He laughed in return and then became serious.

"Pam, I'm so sorry," he said gently, patting my shoulder. "I wish I could make all this move faster; in fact, I wish I could make it all go away."

# TORN ILLUSIONS

"Me, too," I replied.

"But I can't; you know that."

I nodded. He looked at me with empathy.

"One thing of which you may be sure, we'll face this together. And I'm going to give you the best damned legal support I know how to."

Once again I nodded, not trusting myself to speak. Shortly thereafter, I said goodbye. Despite my efforts I couldn't stop shaking as I left his office and walked to my car. "What is happening to me?" I kept murmuring to myself. "Where else in my body will they find it? When will all this be over?" The implications of the report I had read reverberated in my head as I drove home. Once there, I threw myself onto my bed and sobbed. I realized the answer to the questions I'd asked myself was one I'd heard before.

No one knew.

And finding out might take the rest of my life.

While I was fighting my personal battle, the implant industry had incurred major court losses that year involving multi-million dollar awards, which resulted in a backlash of negative media coverage. Their inability to prove the devices' safety with supportive data added to the manufacturers' difficulties. These soon intensified because of the probability of an FDA restriction on silicone implant use in the near future.

Perhaps because of their unfavorable position, Dow Corning and Heyer-Schulte agreed to a voluntary mediation in settlement of my claim for damages due to my silicone implantation. After notifying Judge Highsmith of our good faith agreement and the mutual postponement of the trial date, arbitration was scheduled. During the period preceding this date, however, Dow Corning and Heyer-Schulte canceled the mediation. My lawyers and I were angered by their refusal to honor our agreement. I felt it was another example of the unfair tactics manufacturers used to delay a public trial. During this time, the legal maneuvering appeared to be endless. So I wouldn't obsess over what I could do nothing about, I spent much time researching, investigating and collecting more data. I learned a great deal about silicone, and the February FDA panel review on the heels of the January moratorium provided another valuable supply of information. The testimony and documents presented during the review yielded a wealth of evidence and seemed to provide strong evidence against the manufacturers.[1]

Upon opening the FDA review session, Commissioner Kessler addressed the reasons for the convening of the advisory panel. He said that the earlier November panel had already reached a conclusion; the manufacturer could not prove that a silicone breast implant was a safe product. Commissioner Kessler stated that the issue now was whether or not the devices should remain on the market due to a public health need despite the panel's determination of unproven product safety. He referred to the new information received by the agency after the November 1991 review, which he said had "amplified our concerns" over the reliability of the medical device. Five, three-inch binders containing this data were placed before each panel member. This evidence as to silicone's harm would not be studied or reviewed.

Kessler stated his initial consideration: "One of the things that concern[s] me most is that the breast implants may rupture, leak or bleed more frequently than we had originally thought. We had been told these were rare events."[2] In fact, the newly available information reported the occurrences of rupture to be more than ten times the number previously assumed by the FDA to be accurate. Asymptomatic ruptures were estimated at five percent, which indicated that a great number of implant patients will experience "silent" ruptures (ones undetected by either the physician or patient). Symptomatic ruptures were estimated at another five percent. The two groups, which do not overlap, total 100,000 per one million women who are expected to exhibit, as Dr. Sidney Wolfe explained to the panel, "serious or potentially serious complications."[3] The amount of silicone-gel lost through intact implant shells, by the bleed process, had also been miscalculated. Radiologist Dr. Kathleen Harris of the University of Pittsburgh Medical School stated that gel leakage, which is detectable in lymph nodes, occurs in "100 percent of the cases."[4]

FDA officials presented another concern about implant rupture and gel bleed; the possibility of variations in the silicone gel's solidity. "For example," Dr. Alan Andersen pointed out, "consistency of the gel reportedly varied from batch to batch, and the gel formulation may have changed over time to make it more fluid."[5] He described the fluctuations of one manufacturer's gel to be only borderline between a fluid and gel state. (Understandably, the gel's fluidity probably will facilitate the migration of the silicone.) In addition, the FDA had received evidence that the gel had the ability to cause a swelling of the implants' envelope when it seeps into and interacts with the shell. This results in a reduction of the implant's strength by as much as thirty-three percent over a one year period.[6] The absorption of water and lipids into the implant contributes to the swelling of the shell and places additional pressure upon the device. This rapid and forced weakening of an implant shell signals an earlier and more frequent rupture rate.

Ronald Johnson of the FDA began the review of Dow Corning's internal documents. Dating from 1971 through 1987, the corporate data raised a multitude of questions about the product's safety. Mr. Johnson informed the panel:

> The documents reflect persistent quality control problems,
> as well as concerns about the lack of appropriate
> specifications and overall quality of manufacturing
> operations. They also reveal that in spite of these questions,
> thousands of breast implants were manufactured and
> implanted into women during this time period.[7]

The FDA representative cited many examples from internal documents illustrating the problems in quality control and product testing. For instance, a February 1975 Dow Corning memorandum reported that "envelopes are being manufactured at 1000 per day. Problem: no specifications exist to quality control these bags." Later in April, other corporate records reflected a device rejection rate of at least twenty percent. An official noted, "A large number of people spent a lot of time discussing envelope quality. We ended up saying it was good enough, while looking at the gross, thin spots and flaws in the form of significant bubbles."[8] Subsequent research showed that "bubbles," or weak spots, were detectable in approximately seventeen percent of all implants placed in women.

Dow Corning's reports which were reviewed by the panel seemed to indicate that implant rupture was a much more common occurrence than earlier figures indicated. One of the memorandums described a physician's negative experience. "Upon removal, the prosthesis was partially empty of gel, and what was there was extremely fluid and oozed out of the prosthesis and the surrounding tissue." Also, many company salesmen relayed surgeons' complaints. One reported that an implant ruptured in a physician's hand during surgery while a second implant leaked after autoclaving. Another salesman wrote of ruptures occurring at "an inordinate rate." In December 1977, four physicians informed Dow Corning of a rupture rate of eleven to thirty-two percent.[9] Well into 1978, salesmen continued to report numerous grievances to officials concerning the "excessive rupture rate." There was strong evidence that by 1981, the company's clinical investigator had repeatedly reported these quality control problems. A 1983 internal document cautioned that "the safety of the gel cannot be based on its containment in the shell."[10]

The FDA's examination of Dow Corning studies further illustrated the gel consistency problems. A physician's letter complained that an implant "had gel which literally ran to the floor. We all observed it. It was far from cohesive, having the consistency of fifty weight motor oil."[11] Another physician wrote about "spontaneous, unexplained rupture, inconsistency of shell thickness and gel consistency."[12] These internal documents showed evidence of the seriousness of an implant's bleed of silicone gel. In all regards, it appeared uncontrollable. One study determined, "Gel bleed would have to be reduced by some other means or by new development effort." A memorandum written by company salesman Bob Schnabel indicated not only the implant's leakage of silicone, but also an awareness of its harmfulness. He wrote:

> It has been brought to my attention that this particular lot
> was put on the market with prior knowledge of the bleed
> problem.... To put a questionable lot... on the market is
> inexcusable. I don't know who is responsible for this
> decision, but it has to rank right up

there with the Pinto gas tank.[13]

The Dow Corning employee's sage comparison of the marketing of silicone breast implants to that of the Ford Pinto, which had a defective and explosive gas tank, pointed to the element of greed versus respect for human life and its loss that seems to motivate the decisions of many who profit from others' naiveté.

Dow Corning salesmen repeatedly reported grievances about the devices' objectionable bleed defect. Some sent memorandums detailing the implants' tendency to bleed in their display cases and become oily after being handled. One salesman stated that the implants "bleed profusely after they have been flexed vigorously."[14] When the complaints continued, a large task force finally met to review the matter. One member suggested reformulation of the gel. This was vetoed. In the end, the company decided there wasn't enough evidence and informed neither physicians nor patients of the many reports on the bleed problem.

Some important sources have reported that several instructions were issued to salesmen: instructions on how to clean the implants with soap or alcohol before showing the product to physicians. Next, how to discuss the device without mentioning the bleed defect and how to limit their manipulation of the devices. Finally, it was noted that the implants' silicone oil became noticeable the day after the device was manipulated, thus making it obvious why it wouldn't be noticed in the operating room. Of course, by the next day, the defect would be inconspicuously concealed in the patient's chest.[15] To me, the horror of it is that, with that secret locked safely inside women's bodies, the silicone could then soundlessly leak, seep and migrate undetected.

The advisory panel's review of corporate documents also included a 1977 Dow Corning document (previously under protective order). To me it was astounding. It would seem that a doctor (his name was deleted) had contacted company officials to communicate his interest in obtaining gel-bleed study data. The document discussed what approach to the letter the company should employ. It stated,

Currently, our most applicable date has been generated by [blank]. However, Sue feels that this data should be reproduced before it is even considered for release.... Any general release of this data could be misinterpreted or misconstrued, and could result in severe repercussions in the public sector. However, I still believe that Dow Corning should convey the impression [to the doctor] that we are indeed working in this area. [16]

The alleged desire to camouflage the gel-bleed defect, if true, would have been based upon two important points: First, the patent for the breast implant stated that the gel would be contained in the envelope.[17] Second, the early reports discussing the danger of uncontained silicone in the body (see Chapter Four). Thomas Talcott, a former high-level Dow Corning technical engineer, recognized these dangers. He left the company in 1976 after determining: "Trauma would allow the non-retrievable fluid gel to pass into tissue planes to expose women's bodies to a lifetime of interaction with a likely toxic, dangerous substance." Mr. Talcott was present at the February review and recited his prior court testimony. He stated that "all parties had agreed in that time frame that injectable silicone fluid should not be injected into breast tissue."[18]

The Dow Corning device, once in place, subjected women's breasts to the same substance that had earlier destroyed the breast anatomy of laboratory animals. This information was not conveyed to surgeons or patients. Dr. R. LeVier of Dow Corning has acknowledged that silicone gel, which has been in use since 1975, is ninety percent liquid silicone by weight. Under oath, he has declared the gel implant to be "nothing more than a delivery system for liquid silicone."[19]

Information came out during panel discussions that Dow Corning was asked prior to the February 1992 hearing if the company had ever conducted or witnessed studies showing silicone's stimulation of the immune system. Dow Corning denied both charges. When the existence, as well as the results, of their 1974 study (Chapter Four) became unexpectedly public, the company then stated there was evidence of silicone's immuno-enhancing properties. The conclusion unequivocally stated, "We have data indicating that organo-silicone compounds can stimulate the immune response."[20]

Oven temperatures play a critical role in the process that heats liquid silicone to its gel state. Recent news articles have reported that charts of recorded oven temperatures and substituted replacements over a period of years may not have been reported correctly.[21] Dr. Wolfe of PCHRG verified the importance of oven temperatures. "Depending on what the temperature is, you're going to create different kinds of chemicals. There may be more toxic substances in the gel when it is finished, and it would seem criminal to me to play around with the cooking process."[21]

Dr. Pierre Blais, who has spent years examining retrieved implants, anticipated such a discovery. *The Wall Street Journal* quoted Dr. Blais, who stated, "This is exactly what we suspected for years."[21] He suggested that the resulting variations in the gel may explain why the implants of one manufacturing series were "violently" reactive in some patients and not others. Dr. Blais was also suspicious that oven temperature fluctuations were not the only manufacturing irregularities to have existed. During a January 1993 telephone conversation, Dr. Blais told me that he has observed disparities in the formulation of both the gel and the shell, indicating that the company may not have adhered to standardized formula procedures.

The panel review of internal documents continued to furnish evidence of the lack of safety data. Although evidence revealed that many Dow Corning officials had expressed their concern for years, the inadequacies of the devices were never rectified. In 1975, six months before marketing a new type of silicone implant, A. H. Rathjen, Chairman of the Mammary Task Force, posed the question, "Of absolute and primary importance—will the new gel cause a bleed-through which will make these products unacceptable?"

Other technical advisors had reported the nonexistence of gel bleed tests; however, studies of the new gel that did begin were prematurely terminated. A 1976 memorandum from Mr. Rathjen registered extreme concern. "We are engulfed in unqualified speculation," he wrote. "Nothing to date is truly quantitative. Is there something in the implant that migrates out or off the mammary prosthesis? Yes or no!" A myriad of reports were collected later that year from physicians who had confirmed, through their own patients' experiences, silicone's migration with resulting inflammation in exposed tissues following a short period of implantation. Once again, Mr. Rathjen wrote, "I have proposed again and again that we must begin an in-depth study of our gel, envelope and bleed problem." He also noted that "capsular contracture isn't the only problem. Time is going to run out for us if we don't get underway."[22] Mr. Rathjen, though eagerly requesting the gel study, had himself ordered the length of the studies reduced from ninety to eighty days.[23]

Into the 1980's, the admonitions of company officials went unaddressed and unanswered. A 1983 report implored, "Only inferential data exists. . . . I must strongly urge that Bill's group be given an approval to design and conduct the necessary work to validate that these gels are safe."[24] In 1985, William Boley, the supervisor of Dow Corning's Research and Development Group, expressed the company's need to pursue an adequate study of silicone's cancer-causing potential with a memorandum that closely foretold the future. "Without this testing," he said, "I think we have excessive personal and corporate liability."[25] He also advised the company to warn the public of possible immune disorders.

Nevertheless, Dow Corning refused to enact what many, including me, consider proper and adequate safety testing. Ester Rome of the Boston Women's Health Book Collective and a member of the FDA breast implant force, has stated, when citing 'reliable sources' that "the studies performed by Dow Corning were specifically orchestrated to be poorly conducted."[26] In the event of negative findings, the company could disclaim and confute their own test results.

Dow Corning is not the only company to be singled out. There is much evidence that other implant manufacturers did nothing about investigating implant-related problems, though there were reports of ruptures, bleed, gel inconsistency and silicone migration. As my investigations continued, I spoke to plaintiff attorney Randolph Smith of Dothan, Alabama, about the 1991 Toole versus Heyer-Schulte case: I learned that among the most damaging evidence presented at trial were letters of complaint Heyer-Schulte received throughout the years. The Toole trial resulted in an award of $5.4 million against this manufacturer. (The plaintiff was offered only a $20,000 settlement before trial.) When I spoke to Dr. Blais, who has studied all the implant models, he described the Heyer-Schulte implant as one of the worst. "The Heyer-Schulte implants," he has said, "would cleave in half and spill the contents, producing gross deformities."[27] He added that many serious health problems were associated with this particular product.

The shortage of safety data among the majority of implant manufacturers echoes that of Dow Corning. Dr. Blais, who testified before the December 18, 1990 Congressional Subcommittee hearing, stated at the time that the testing conducted by the entire implant industry over the past thirty years had been "trivial, if not totally irrelevant." Larry Charfois, an attorney representing the plaintiffs in a breast-implant litigation, has also stated that "nobody at 3M, McGhan or Heyer-Schulte did any testing to see about the systemic effects" of silicone.[28] Jan Varner, president of McGhan, acknowledged that the company "relied very heavily" on the Dow Corning study material.[29] Of course, this reliance occurred despite the fact that Dow Corning's testing, while insufficient, had proven silicone to be a questionable substance. (There is a similarity among the implant manufacturers' products. Many toxic-chemical components of both the shell and the gel exist in silicone implants, regardless of their make or model.)

As to the industry's knowledge of risks and lack of safety data Attorney Dan Bolton's 1991 letter to Commissioner Kessler stated that "considerable evidence was presented at trial that Dow was aware of the risks of silicone as early as the 1960s. . . [while] Dow's own product literature represented that breast implants were safe for long term use by women."[30] During testimony given before the February review, Mr. Bolton made reference to a brochure entitled, "Facts You Should Know About Your New Look," which Dow Corning distributed directly to women during the 1970s. The literature, he said, had falsely stated that "implants were completely safe, 'well-tolerated' by the body, and 'based on laboratory findings, should last a lifetime.'" However, Dow Corning's 1991 product literature later conceded that, contrary to its previous claim, the life-expectancy of the implant was "unpredictable." The revised brochure further disclosed that "the long-term physiological effects of uncontained silicone are currently unknown."[31] In this time period, the Public Citizens Health Resource Group filed labeling violations against Bioplasty, Mentor and McGhan, as well as Dow Corning, for distributing fallacious and misleading information to prospective implant recipients. This false and misleading information no doubt deprived many vulnerable women of their right to be informed and give informed consent.

Ester Rome of Boston Women's Health Book Collection told the panel that informed consent involves "knowing the rate of complications or understanding that you are part of an experiment. Neither of these criteria," she pointed out, "have been met in the case of silicone gel-filled implants."

Representative Joan Pitkin of the Maryland State Legislature, who was also present at the panel review, had campaigned for informed consent among implant patients for many years. She described the hostilities surrounding her efforts: "In 1981, I introduced legislation to mandate that brochures be given to anyone choosing breast reconstruction or augmentation. This legislation was opposed by manufacturers and members of the medical community." Representative Pitkin's bill floundered until 1987 when it finally passed. She said that other legislation, designed for the purpose of weakening this new law, was soon introduced, but subsequently defeated. Representative Pitkin continued, "A number of other states attempted similar initiatives, only to fail because of the opposition based on the opinion that disclosure of all risks and complications would have a chilling effect on consumer choice."[32] I feel the industry failed to disclose these problems so as to obscure the many deadly risks and to continue selling what many had to suspect or know was a deadly product.

This seems true in many areas. A review of Dow Corning research on animal studies during the early years uncovers hazards of silicone. The industry had not publicly disclosed its research for over twenty years while marketing the devices. By 1968, tests conducted by Dow Corning had reported gel bleed which resulted in migration, and also the cancer-causing properties of silicone. How could other implant companies, created by former Dow scientists, not know of these dangers?

Included in the 1986 Dow Corning animal study data were tissue examinations of silicone-injected rats and mice. The specimens established silicone's migration to these organs and glands: spleen, liver, kidneys, pancreas, uterus, ovaries, adrenals, small intestine and lymph nodes.[33] Silicone was identified in much of the surrounding fat removed with the tissue samples. Although these results are disturbing, more disturbing is the pronounced incidence of malignant cancer produced in the same rodent studies.[33] Dow Corning scientists reported finding of lymphoma and leukemia in all of the rodents' organs and glands listed above, plus the salivary glands. Samples in some test series provided evidence of coexistent cancer and migrated silicone; these included the spleen, kidney and pancreas. Far worse for the female implant patient, adenocarcinoma, a malignant gland cancer, developed in animals' ovaries and uteruses.[34]

Although the FDA did not present this information to the panel for their review, Dr. Norman Anderson of Johns Hopkins School of Medicine, confronted Dr. LeVier of Dow Corning with these same studies during the panel discussions. Levier then stated that the Dow Corning data report of an eighty percent incidence of lymphoma in the mice had been discredited under audit and was determined instead to be a one hundred percent incidence of cancer having occurred in the laboratory animals.[35] Dr. Sidney Wolfe, Director of PCHRG, later told the panel that Dow Corning's silicone gel had also "induced highly-malignant sarcomas when injected into rats."[36]

The FDA's review of the Dow Corning animal studies also included further discussions of the early knowledge of gel migration, which company researchers reaffirmed in the 1970s. One 1975 study of a new gel formulation again showed silicone's travel throughout the bodies of test animals. In spite of this finding, the implants containing the gel formula in question were marketed to the general public. In reference to other radioactive-labelled studies conducted in 1976 and 1977, Mr. McGunagle of the FDA reported that "portions of the liquid silicone component can be distributed throughout the body."[37] Moreover, it was not possible to recover all of the gel loss. A 1978 rat study determined that "eighty-four days after the injection of gel into the rat, it was physically possible to recover only fifty-three percent of the injected gel weight." One company official concluded that "the apparent disappearance of fifty percent of the gel from the injection site is of concern." A rabbit study involving the implantation of the prosthesis also reported that only half of the gel could be recovered after eighty-four days. The fibrous capsule, described by Dr. Blais during panel testimony "as the only barrier between physiologic and biologic catastrophe," was shown to be an ineffective protection against the gel's migration. A Dow Corning researcher noted that "in rabbits at six months after implantation, the gel mass is fragmented by tissue ingrowth . . . rarely had the consulting pathologist reported the presence of the gel at the original implantation side." An assessment of the rat and rabbit gel recovery studies prompted the researcher to write, "These two pieces of animal data cast suspicion on the ability of a fibrous tissue capsule to prevent distribution of gel to other parts of the body."[38]

The fibrous tissue ingrowth, which entirely penetrated the gel mass while breaking and partitioning it into smaller masses, both complicated and inhibited gel recovery. The studies confirmed that "varying degrees of tissue ingrowth can take place with free silicone in the body." The researcher reported that "the portioning phenomenon also greatly increases the surface area of gel exposed to tissues. This increased tissue area may result in more rapid removal of the gel from the implant site by phagocytic cells." The author's conclusion stated, "It is reasonable to postulate a similar phenomenon may occur in humans."[39]

The study of the migration of silicone in the bodies of test animals resulted in other disturbing laboratory findings as well. Dr. John Langone of the FDA reviewed the early evidence of extensive silicone-induced chronic foreign body reaction, inflammation and organ damage, which developed in the test animals. One of the 1968 rodent studies reported a fifty to ninety percent occurrence of liver and splenic "abnormalities" and "chronic kidney inflammation."[40]

Granulomas, fat necrosis (death of cells), adrenal hypervolemia (increased volume) and gland hyperplasias (enlargements) were also present. This agreed with my own medical experience, as I had suffered pituitary gland enlargement following my implant operation. It didn't recede until five years after the implants were removed. The animal studies I read determined that a seventy percent incidence of glomerular (kidney) lesions in the mice indicated an immunologic response. Vacuolated cells, which are ones containing holes, were another common finding and compatible with the presence of silicone in these cells.

In studies on apes conducted in the late 1960s, Dow Corning pathologists observed more hyperplasia, kidney abnormalities, lung edema and chronic stomach inflammation among these animals. Vacuolated cells were located in the breast tissue of three of four primates and were even found prevalent in the lungs.[41] The animal data also reported extraordinary occurrences of necrosis of the liver. Dr. Marc Lappé, a panel consultant, stated that researchers at the Huntington Laboratory reported this specific organ damage to be "biologically significant and not explained by the presence of tumors or by the presence of anything but your [the manufacturer's] gels in these animals."[42]

Silicone research of the same time period involved dogs, a substantial number of them developed chronic thyroiditis, which is an inflammation of the thyroid gland. In press statements, Dr. Lappé has referred to the fact that the 1974 study should have been "a three-bar storm warning" that a leaking breast implant might similarly enhance an immune response in women.[43] When laboratory dogs were studied later in the 1970s, most of these subjects again exhibited inflammatory reactions, and one dog died of "unknown causes."[44] In the case of thirty-eight beagles, these silicone-tested animals developed an incredible 200 percent higher spleen weight than did the control dogs, or untreated (non-implanted) animals used as a basis for comparison in laboratory testing. During the panel review, Dr. Langone discussed the abnormal tissue weights and their importance in relationship to the immunologic effects of silicone. He reported that "these abnormalities are, in our [the FDA's] opinion, cause for concern."[45]

This, I believe, is an understatement, for the abnormalities are more than a "concern." A 200 percent higher spleen weight should be considered a cause for alarm.

During the review of the animal studies, Dr. Lappé further told the panel that "lymph node enlargements" existed "in virtually every animal study."[46] It was also made known in panel testimony (and supported by court evidence) that Dow Corning had known of silicone's migration throughout the lymphatic system to various organs of the immune system as early as 1972.[47] Concerning the FDA's appraisal of the Dow Corning animal data, which revealed silicone's effects on the immune system in guinea pigs and rats, Dr. Langone stated the FDA's conclusion:

> We agree that certain silicones tested can indeed act as
> adjuvants to enhance the antibody response to a standard
> antigen in experimental animals. The number of silicones,
> however, with adjuvant activity may be greater than the
> authors conclude.[48]

One cannot dispute the relevance of this animal testing. It would be foolish to believe that human beings are in some way unique from all other mammals and thereby excluded from the potential for silicone-induced illness and abnormalities suffered by these laboratory animals. If animal study did not hold serious implications for human illness, it would not be an important and accepted preliminary study to human research trials. After a review of both the animal studies and the FDA's own conclusions, I felt anyone would feel that human beings would have similar reactions. To me it is incomprehensible, in light of the evidence of the dangers of silicone shown by animal testing, that the industry did not curtail silicone implant manufacturing. Instead, according to the corporate documents I reviewed, Dow Corning, the largest implant producer and distributor who many other companies emulated, stopped testing the silicone. While manufacturers counted their profits, women like me paid the price—a far dearer one than we could ever have expected.

The next area I studied was that of silicone as the cause of illnesses. I found that in February of 1992 the FDA panel reviewed various aspects of the silicone implant's potential for causing human illness. Evidence of chronic foreign body reaction and inflammation in association with human silicone exposure was presented, and the possibilities for resulting illness were discussed. Dr. Kathleen Harris of the University of Pittsburgh Medical School provided a demonstration of silicone lymphadenopathy which was represented by a giant foreign body cell holding a globule of silicone within its body. She also discussed silicone migration to lymph nodes as a result of gel bleed through intact shells.[49] Dr. Judy Destouet of the Washington University School of Medicine in St. Louis, showed mammographic evidence of silicone granulomas and gel migration to the lymph nodes.[50]

Dr. Lori Love of the FDA defined the granuloma formations as a distinctive pattern of inflammation occurring after exposure to materials that cannot be broken down by the body. The cells in the granulomas may themselves induce illness, for they are able to secrete substances known as cytokines, which have wide-ranging effects upon the body (Chapter VIII). Several clinicians and physicians attested to the capability of the pro-inflammatory cytokines to cause symptoms of illness.[51] It was suggested that some of the flu-like symptoms experienced by many implant patients could be attributed to the presence of the secreting cells within the silicone granulomas.[52] (Medical evidence that became available in 1993 supports this concern and is discussed in Chapter IX).

During the panel's review of the inflammatory illness aspect of silicone implantation, Dr. Norman Anderson presented his theory regarding the attempt to place an implanted woman's illness into a known, existing disease category. He suggested that in the process "a chronic illness caused by chronic inflammation" may have possibly been overlooked. Dr. Bernard Patten of Baylor College of Medicine also considered the foreign body inflammation to be pertinent. In quoting Voltaire, Dr. Patten stressed that the concern was an ageless one:

> 'The interaction of the human body with a foreign
> substance.' That's what we're talking about. If you have a
> body that evolved over three million years, [sic] to reject
> foreign material, and you introduce a substance like

silicone, or something similar to silicone—silicate or silicone
dioxide—and I have a feeling the breast implant also
contains catalyst and a whole bunch of foreign materials,
you have to expect a reaction. It's only logical.[53]

Dr. Patten's anxiety about the foreign matter contained in any
silicone implant is justified. Although the virulent nature of many
chemicals found in the implants are currently unknown, others are
well known to cause human illness.

The panel listened to evidence about the presence of these
harmful chemicals as another aspect of silicone implant-related illness.
David McGunagle of the FDA cited a study that determined that a
mixture containing as many as thirty different chemicals is released by
both the gel and the shell. He said that most of the chemicals remain
unidentified, but "of the few chemicals that were identified and
qualified, one is of particular interest."[54] The chemical he made
reference to is octomethylcyclotetra-siloxane, more familiarly known
as D4. Mr. McGunagle stated that the identification of D4 from both
the gel and the shell had "potential significance" in the association
between silicone and immune disorders. In fact, an FDA "Talk Paper"
later discussed Dow Corning studies conducted in 1993 that
established the silicone gel to be an adjuvant, which produced a
"strong antibody response" (Chapter VIII). Autoimmune illness could
be a possible consequence of exposure to this gel.

Chemical agents are presently *linked* to many autoimmune
illnesses. Numerous drugs contain these agents; several examples are
Hydralazine, Procainamide, Neomycin and D-penicillamine.[55] Some
types of Lupus reactions are also drug related, and a few chemicals
associated with scleroderma (a thickening and tightening of the skin)
are Spanish toxic oil, trichloroethylene and vinyl chloride.[56] Of great
significance to the implant patient, it is important to note that the
agent silica is known to induce scleroderma. (Much available evidence
also links silica to rheumatoid arthritis.[57]) The silica/scleroderma
connection is especially interesting because although scleroderma is
one of the rarest of the autoimmune illnesses, this illness is frequently
reported in patients who have silicone implants.

# TORN ILLUSIONS

Silica, silastic and silicone are organic compounds that replace carbon with silicon. A 1993 medical journal publication provided the first dramatic "demonstration of the spread of silicon-containing substance from silicone gel-filled implants to actual sites of connective-tissue disease."[58] In three cases, silicon was identified within the tissues "in association with evidence of connective-tissue disease." The study of one implant patient, who developed scleroderma following her operation, reported that "silicon had been detected within the involved skin, but not within the uninvolved skin." The authors of the article maintained:

> The presence of silicon-containing material within sites of
> connective-tissue disease supports a role for silicon in the
> origin of such conditions in patients with silicone-gel
> implants. All patients with connective-tissue disease should
> be questioned about exposure to various forms of silicon. In
> those patients with known exposure, tissue specimens
> should be examined carefully for silicon-containing material
> and, if found, the source should be removed.

The authors stated that after reporting the findings of this research, three additional breast implant patients were found to have silicon present within sites of their connective-tissue disease.

As I revealed in Chapter Four, many researchers have long stated their concern that silicone may be converted by the body into silica. I discussed this issue with Dr. Blais, and he explained that when burned, silicone oil breaks down to silicone dioxide, which is "the skeleton" of silicone. For example, if a bovie, a high frequency surgical cauterizing knife, comes in contact with body tissue containing deposited silicone oil, the tissue turns white. The eventual breakdown of silicone to silica within the body would be a more debatable issue were it not for the discovery that the manufacturers have intentionally included silica as a filler in silicone gel-fill, as well as for use as a fortifier in the implant shell.[59] According to Dr. Blais, all implant shells, including the saline implant shell, have a thirty percent silica component.[60] In panel testimony, Dr. Patten also referred to both the presence of silica and its bearing upon immune illnesses reported today. He stated:

> The most important things you've heard this morning was
> that fume silica is actually added to the elastomer shell. . . .
> Now that is a bad actor in medicine. We know it's an
> adjuvant; we know it's responsible for silicosis. . . . This is a
> well known adjuvant. In addition, silicon causes
> cancer—asbestos is a generic term for silicates. Asbestos
> causes cancer of the lung, and mesothelioma, and there's no
> dispute about that. So chemistry is destiny. If you're putting
> this material—injecting it in, or putting it in the bag that
> leaks or bleeds—you have to run into trouble and I think
> that's what we're seeing.[61]

I agree with Dr. Patten's assessment. Furthermore, I consider it a heinous offense to have included a deadly substance of such notoriety in a product that would be implanted in millions of women.

More studies of many chemical, environmental agents, and their relationship to human illness, are now under way. Dr. Joseph Bellanti, former president of the American College of Allergy and Immunology, stated that this organization is in the process of reviewing many of the issues concerning the effects of chemical agents upon the immune system. Referring to the issue of silicone's involvement in the immune system, Dr. Bellanti suggested that one possibility may be silicone's reactivation of latent viruses lingering, which are now linked to autoimmune illness.[62] If this is the case, it would then constitute yet another cause of illness.

Dr. Noel Rose of the Allergy and Immunology department of Johns Hopkins School of Medicine, also spoke before the advisory panel. Hired by Mentor Corporation to represent the manufacturer during the panel's review of the silicone/autoimmune illness connection, Dr. Rose discussed several possible immune system responses to silicone. He said that "human hypersensitivity" was one possible response, but there is "virtually no evidence from humans that such reactions occur."[63] I feel this is not so, as my own allergic reaction to silicone and those of women in many other reported cases seems evidence enough of a human hypersensitivity to silicone. Dr. Rose did make a statement with which I agree, however. He stated that prolonged exposure to silicone when in a hypersensitive state with antigenic response may result in a second immune occurrence, known as immune complex disease. In these diseases, antigens and antibodies collide and join together to form large complexes that "clog" the lymphatic system. Lupus is an example of an immune complex disease that is also an autoimmune illness due to the production of autoantibodies.

The ability of silicone to induce human hypersensitivity has obvious consequences. Just as my body responded to silicone as an antigenic agent, it is likely that others would have the same response. Dr. Ira Finegold has determined that "patch tests indicate reactions to silicone in almost twenty percent of implant patients." A 1994 paper with Dr. Finegold's authorization cited a 26 percent positive reaction.[64] The result of these allergic reactions, as supported by Dr. Rose, can be silicone-associated immune complex disease.

The panel studied autoimmune illness as a third possible immune occurrence. In pointing out the FDA's concern over the clinical evidence of autoimmune/connective tissue disease in association with silicone breast implants, Dr. Alan Andersen of the FDA stated, "Since our last meeting, we have become aware of more clinical reports of implant patients with a wide variety of autoimmune-like symptoms. . . . For the first time, we've heard of neurological problems in breast implant patients who also exhibit autoimmune-like symptoms."[65] Dr. Mary B. Jacobs of the FDA began the panel's review of the autoimmune illness issue with an update of a preliminary screening of physicians, which was conducted by the FDA's Center for Biologic Evaluation of Research. The screening obtained responses from twenty-six physicians, most of whom were rheumatologists. The majority of the physicians contacted by the agency were currently treating at least one to three implant patients with the reported illness, and eight physicians followed ten to two hundred and fifty such patients.

Dr. Frederick Miller, a rheumatologist with the FDA, discussed silicone breast implant-associated illnesses: rheumatic disorders, which are a family of more than one hundred illnesses involving the connective tissues of the body. This type of disease can effect the bones, joints, muscles, tendons, ligaments, skin and covering tissue. Therefore, they are referred to as connective-tissue diseases. The diffusive connective-tissue disorders are distinguished by systemic inflammation and autoimmune features. When antibodies, which are circulating blood proteins that protect against infection, react against one's own tissue, they become known as autoantibodies. This is one feature of autoimmune disease. Lymphocytes, white blood cells, may also become self-reactive and result in injury to a person's tissue and body. This is considered to be another autoimmune feature of rheumatic illness.

Due to the variety of symptoms that often overlap, many rheumatologists place patients into diagnostic categories that follow recognizable patterns. To lessen confusion, a list of criteria has been established by some rheumatologists to aid in the diagnosis of the rheumatic diseases. A number of patients have a combination of symptoms and laboratory abnormalities which do not meet any specified criteria. They are often referred to as having mixed connective-tissue disease. Some patients exhibit autoantibodies; others do not.

Rheumatoid arthritis, the most frequently diagnosed connective-tissue disease, may range from a mild condition to a severe, incapacitating and life-endangering illness. Lupus erythematosus is not as common and involves an inflammation of any part of the body. It is characterized by a facial rash over the nose and cheeks. Systemic sclerosis, another connective-tissue illness, is considered a rare disorder. The dominant feature of sclerosis is scleroderma, a thickening and tightening of the skin. Although the causes of connective-tissue disease are unknown, Dr. Miller stated that environmental factors may influence susceptibility to this disorder.[66]

The advisory panel heard the testimony of three rheumatologists. The first speaker, Dr. Frank Vasey of the University of South Florida College of Medicine in Tampa, who has significant clinical experience with the reported rheumatic illnesses of implant patients, presented his findings to the assembly. One of his first patients who exhibited silicone-associated illness was a Japanese woman. Following breast injections of silicone, she developed scleroderma-like symptoms, which the medical literature describes as being silicone related. A second patient, one with silicone implants, also suffered scleroderma-like symptoms and only improved after her explantation. A third breast implant patient, whose illness resembled Lupus erythematosus, responded in the same manner. Upon the removal of her implants, Dr. Vasey stated that she is in "complete remission and feels 100 percent normal." After presenting these cases to the 1990 National Rheumatology meeting as well as to a public FDA hearing, women learned of Dr. Vasey's interest in the silicone issue and soon arrived at his clinic. At the time of this panel review, 300 implant patients were under his care.

Two of Dr. Vasey's patients' implants ruptured at a precise recorded time. In both cases the implants were accidentally punctured by the general surgeons during breast biopsies; neither surgeon removed the prostheses. Dr. Vasey showed slides of a large erythematous (bruised area) which occurred as the silicone traveled down the chest of one of the patients. Soon, symptoms of myalgias and arthralgias, which are respectively muscle and joint pain, developed, as did chronic fatigue and swollen lymph nodes. Dr. Vasey determined that many of his patients become quickly symptomatic after a rupture or some other form of implant trauma. Although a number of women experience pain immediately after implantation and an early progression of silicone illness symptoms as I did, for others there is a latency period of as many as nine years before silicone illness symptoms begin to develop. Dr. Vasey reported that a small number of patients have implants on only one side and that he has been "impressed" because they exhibit "increased prevalence of symtomatology on the implant side." Dr. Vasey described one colleague's patient who "had a left-sided breast implant, and had more skin tightening in her scleroderma syndrome on the left chest wall and in the left arm."[67]

Dr. Vasey classified the chronic flu-like illness of implant patients, who experience fibromyalgia, polyarthralgia, lymphadenopathy and swollen joints, as "atypical rheumatic disease syndromes." He noted that some patients do, however, exhibit "terribly devastating" scleroderma. Dr. Vasey has found a reasonably high prevalence of ANA, or antinuclear antibodies, yet his patients improved by a rate of seventy percent after the devices' removal. He concluded the following, "It is my feeling that unusual constellations of signs and symptoms do indeed reflect immune response to the silicone particles."[68]

Dr. Vasey, as do many other rheumatologists, also treats saline implant patients with similar associated illnesses. I am acquainted with one of his patients who developed a severe illness following her saline implantation. Another personal friend is also recovering from an autoimmune illness related to the placement of her saline implants. Both of these women were greatly incapacitated, and after explantation, both improved significantly.

During a recent conversation with Dr. Vasey, he asked if I had experienced an initial worsening of symptoms before my progress began. I replied that I had. He explained that this was a frequent occurrence among patients who have silicone breast implants removed. Although this post-explantation route to recovery is generally not understood, it may be due to a release and mobilization of silicone and other implant-associated chemicals.

Dr. Steven Weiner, Chief of Rheumatology at the University of California at Los Angeles, gave the next presentation. Having followed numerous implant patients since 1981, he was one of the first rheumatologists to suspect an association between silicone implants and connective-tissue disease. Dr. Weiner prefers the term "CSA" (chronic silicone arthropathy) to define implant patients who display myalgias, arthalgias or neuralgias that remain undiagnosed and unresponsive to therapy after a one year period. He stated that it was unusual for a physician to see a non-implant patient for a year without determining a diagnosis of their illness or achieving a response to treatment. He does not include any implant patient who has a "known rheumatic disease" in the CSA category.

Dr. Weiner related the results of a survey that he and his colleagues conducted through the United Scleroderma Foundation's newsletter. From the responses of over twenty-five women who developed distinct scleroderma after silicone implantation, fourteen reported improvement upon explantation. Dr. Weiner emphasized the importance of these findings as scleroderma usually does not improve. He referred to Dr. Metgers, a national clinical authority who "flatly states systemic sclerosis does not improve."

Dr. Weiner discussed a study of fifty CSA patients. Their symptoms developed within two to twenty-two years following their implantations. He found frequent ruptures of the devices, and seventy-five percent of his patients had experienced capsular contracture. He also reported the occurrence of lymphadenopathy, fatigue, flu-like symptoms and Raynaud's and Scheie's syndrome, and at least half of a group of 150 women tested were ANA positive. Dr. Weiner told the panel that he has come across saline implant patients who become symptomatic after implantation. On average, ten out of fifteen of his implant patients have improved after a removal of their implants. Dr. Weiner concluded that CSA patients do not meet any criteria for "known rheumatic illness" and do not respond to "standard treatment." They have a "higher incidence" of "lymphadenopathy, capsular contracture, and implant rupture" without "other medical explanations for symptoms" except "prolonged exposure to silicone," and respond favorably to explantation.[69]

Dr. Harry Spiera of Mount Sinai Medical Center in New York, was the third rheumatologist who spoke before the advisory panel. He became interested in silicone-associated illnesses after reading medical literature, and in particular a 1984 paper by Dr. Kumagai published in *Arthritis and Rheumatism*, which described a group of implant patients resembling those Dr. Weiner saw in his own practice.[70] He was "struck" by the observation that out of 112 consecutive patients, five were implant patients who showed up without a referral. Dr. Spiera published research concerning implant-related disorders in 1988.[71] At the time of the FDA review, he had followed fifty-five implant patients with connective-tissue disease.

In his presentation, Dr. Spiera described the illnesses he found in his implant patients. He could not identify the diseases of six women who experienced myalgias, arthralgias, and low-grade fevers; these were probable ANA positive. He diagnosed four patients with Sjogren's syndrome. Three others he regarded as having adjuvant disease with silicone present "in different parts of their body as manifested by swelling elsewhere, and [who] had positive biopsies of lymph nodes."[72] They also exhibited "fevers, arthralgias, myalgias and malaise." Three patients had symptoms of arthritis, and one woman suffered a "sarcoid-like disease" with fever, lymphadenopathy and granulomas. Two of five patients with fibromyalgia were ANA positive. One patient was characteristic of Lupus erythematosus, and two others typified dermatomyositis. Of special significance was the fact that several of Dr. Spiera's patients had silicone chin implants. One breast implant patient displayed facial swelling, which Dr. Spiera said resembled scleroderma without other characteristics of the disease. (Like myself, many implanted women experience this same facial swelling.) One of his scleroderma patients visited two medical centers for consultation before going to Dr. Spiera. She had asked the other physicians if her scleroderma could be related to the implant. They all said no. When the woman declined treatment and subsequently consulted Dr. Spiera, he advised her that she "might want to take the breast implants out." After a removal of the implants, she has made "definite improvement," which has continued for four years.

Dr. Spiera went on to tell about several tragic deaths. One occurred in a patient with aggressive dermatomyositis who chose not to have the implants removed. Another patient, whose husband gave her implants for her fiftieth birthday, developed a "febrile illness" two months later. Her health rapidly deteriorated, and although the implants were later removed, she eventually died from her illness. A third death occurred in a young patient who experienced scleroderma post-implantation. She initially refused to have the implants removed, but she became progressively worse and finally underwent an explantation; the woman died shortly afterwards with her two-year-old child in her lap. Dr. Spiera concluded that if an association between the deaths and the silicone implants is "real," then it is "an extremely serious one." He was also "most frightened" by the "incredible incidence of scleroderma."[73]

Following Dr. Spiera, Dr. Bernard Patten, a neurologist at Baylor College of Medicine in Dallas, discussed the evidence of the involvement of the central nervous system in autoimmune illnesses of implant patients. Dr. Patten had treated implant patients with serious neurological complications and disease for five years. His study of those patients resulted in a paper he presented to the American Neurological Association in 1991. Dr. Patten focused on two of the many implant patients that he and his Baylor colleagues had examined. The first patient experienced severe headaches three years after implantation and also developed Parinaud's Syndrome (an inability to look up). He reported that her MRI showed brain lesions indicating multiple sclerosis, but her spinal fluid isolated an elevated protein that is not associated with the multiple sclerosis disease. Soon she became weak and showed hyperactive reflexes. There was a loss of blood supply to several of her fingers. Eventually, gangrene developed in all of her fingers, and one finger later required amputation. Talking about these sad occurrences, Dr. Patten remarked, "We didn't know what this was. It doesn't resemble any known neurological disease, but our Japanese colleagues helped us out with some of the cases they reported in medical literature that were due to silicone injections, and we thought we were dealing with silicone adjuvant disease." During the patient's evaluation, Dr. Heggers determined the presence of blood antibodies to silicone. After one woman's implants were removed, both were found to be ruptured in spite of her mammogram showing a normal reading. Dr. Patten stated that other than a few headaches and the loss of her finger, the woman is now completely normal. (As a pertinent example of the pressing need for awareness within the medical community concerning silicone implant-associated disorders, the neurologist who referred this woman to the Baylor physicians had not known that his female patient had breast implants).

The second implant patient Dr. Patten discussed had an illness which bore a resemblance to amyotrophic lateral sclerosis, sometimes called Lou Gehrig's disease. However, when her ruptured implants were removed, Dr. Patten said, "Lo and behold, her so-called amyotrophic lateral sclerosis, a disease that hardly ever or never, in my experience, improves by itself, got better."[74] This woman is still alive after having had her implants removed in 1985. Dr. Patten told the panel that he was presently monitoring seven patients with implants who had this disease.

Dr. Patten also demonstrated the effects of an implant spill with photographic evidence which contradicted a plastic surgeon's claim that escaped silicone could easily be removed. "This is a gigantic mess," he stated. "Look at that gummy mess; in tissue the surgeon will spend hours and hours trying to get it out. It's almost impossible to remove." Dr. Patten further confirmed the bleed of implants. "Just put them on the table for five minutes and then lift them up; you'll see this little greasy oil spot on the bottom, so they all bleed."[75] Then he presented examples of dense, chronic inflammation with classic foreign body giant cells, which included silicone within their centers. Dr. Patten stated that, at the time of each explantation, he conducts muscle and nerve biopsies, also informing the panel that he had provided the FDA with a forty-seven page report profiling the histologic abnormalities of implant patients as determined by the Baylor physicians.

From clinical observations, Dr. Patten found that the illness begins with muscle weakness, fatigue and generalized symptoms. He said:

> This weakness is real. Eventually it begins to have an
> impact on their life. . . . They can't get out of the bathtub.
> They trip and fall. . . . They have trouble brushing their
> teeth. They can't button their clothes. . . . You're talking
> about real weakness.[76]

In tests measuring muscle strength, the patients perform at six to thirty percent of what is expected of women at their ages. Dr. Patten described the "fatigability" of implant patients as common and disabling. He commented, "They'll spend eighteen hours in bed; some of them spend all their time in bed." The symptoms of weakness and fatigue are often followed by myalgias, arthralgias, muscle atrophy and stiffness with Raynaud's and Scheie's syndrome. Dr. Patten has detected sensory loss reflecting the neuropathy; yet patients also have increased reflexes due to nervous system myelopathy (a disease of the myelin which covers the nerves) or develop brain lesions. He reported that his patients have serious short-term memory deficits, not unlike my own earlier memory loss. In one demonstration, Dr. Patten showed the photographic slides of a woman who exhibited a "combination of scleroderma, dermatomyositis and peripheral neuropathy; a very swollen face and swollen lymph nodes. . . ." He asked, "Is someone going to tell me that her body is not reacting to this implant?"[77]

Dr. Patten documented two implant-related deaths at the February 1992 review. However, the number of fatalities has rapidly risen. The Manufacturer Device Reporting Program (MDR) acknowledged eighteen breast implant-associated deaths as of the end of 1992.[78] Although 21,120 implant-related illnesses and injuries were reported at that time, two months later the figures had climbed by 18,000.[79] The 1993 figures, which do not include the physician-reported cases of silicone illness, show an average of 3,390 additional reports per month. Within another two months, a periodic newsletter published by the Coalition of Silicone Survivors (COSS), a support organization, stated MDR figures of 33,825 injuries and twenty-six deaths as of May 19, 1993. This two-month span averaged 2,913 implant injuries per month with eight deaths having occurred in a six month frame. By August 5, 1993, the MDR included another four deaths and 5,336 more injuries. The FDA's estimation of silicone-associated illnesses has quickly become outdated. In fact, the current MDR figures report, as of June 1994, a total of 74,336 injured women and 52 deaths.[80] Due to the industry's history of MDR violations concerning data reported to the FDA, these figures must be labeled conservative and their accuracy considered questionable.

At the end of his speech, Dr. Patten expressed the seriousness of this grim disease:

> Atypical everything. Kidney failure, liver failure and the multifocal, white matter lesions that appeared to be due to vascular involvement, not multiple sclerosis. . . . I've been a neurologist for twenty-five years and I examine in adult neurology for the American Board of Psychiatry in neurology, and I'd have to say that none of these patients fits into a clearly-defined, identifiable, well-known, organized, coherent, known neurological disorder. Each of them has a peculiar or several peculiar features, including a host of abnormal antibodies and abnormalities that we

would identify with that particular illness. . . . So we have solid data that there's no question these people are very sick.[81]

On a daily basis, other physicians and rheumatologists are seeing patients who have implants and have silicone associated disease. If the Japanese experience with breast injections is a harbinger of other women's fate, the number of silicone-implanted women stricken will continue to rise. In fact, it may be years or decades before the true impact of silicone's migration and the subsequent release of toxic chemicals from the gel and shell are fully realized by implant recipients and their children.

Although many questions remain unanswered, much information was revealed during the three-day FDA review. Information about early research studies by Dow Corning and other implant manufacturers which contain an enormous amount of data about the possible injurious nature of silicone implants were studied. Much of it had not been previously released to the FDA, physicians or the women who were to receive the implanted devices. There were discussions and evidence offered about possibly dangerous, poisonous substances added to implant products. Moreover, serious questions were raised about manufacturers' disregard for safety precautions and their inhibiting of testing. The procurement of "protective" and "gag" orders were also addressed (Chapter X). To me, it seems apparent that for decades Dow Corning and other implant companies used and abused their influence and power in order to not be held accountable for any adverse results of implant use.

I feel each and every implant recipient should have the benefit of legal recourse, with or without current existing illness, due solely to a very real possibility, if not probability, that many may suffer implant-related illnesses of some type in the future.

I fervently agree with Representative Pitkin who poignantly stated during panel testimony, "A crime has been perpetrated on these women, and now the manufacturers' cynical lack of concern for today's victims is something you must address—we must all address."[82]

# 7

# NEW DIRECTIONS

After the FDA review session concluded, I felt reenergized and looked forward to the rescheduling of my court date, which had been delayed by Judge Highsmith's reexamination of my case after arbitration. As it had for me, the panel's determinations held particular interest and implication for other women immersed in their own liability legalities. These women had anxiously awaited the outcome of the FDA panel's deliberations in the hopes of finding answers to their own questions concerning implant safety. Media reports on different parts of the hearing, including excerpts from Dow Corning's documents, had fueled public indignation. There was public outcry that the indiscriminate use of silicone implants should no longer continue.

It had been sixteen years since Congress empowered the regulatory agency with the authority to oversee the medical device industry and many years since reports of silicone's danger were circulated. Although it was too late for many women, the FDA advisory panel now recommended the removal of silicone-gel implants from the general market with a virtual ban on their use for cosmetic purposes. Reconstructive implantation would be allowed in mastectomy patients and in women with congenital deformities or traumatic breast injury, but these procedures required a physician's statement claiming that saline implants were not a satisfactory alternative. In these cases, a detailed consent form had to be signed, and all patients enrolled in clinical studies. Regarding cosmetic augmentation with silicone-gel implants, FDA spokeswoman Sharon Snider stated that "only a few women who want them for cosmetic reasons will have access to clinical studies. The numbers would be in the hundreds."[1] The hospitals and plastic surgeons chosen to participate in the clinical trials were to be limited. Although Commissioner Kessler would not issue his final ruling on the panel's directives until April 16th, his approval was anticipated.

In the interim, many women evaluated the ramifications of the silicone breast implant issue. Hundreds of thousands of women had implants themselves. Women without the prostheses had concerns for their friends or family members who were implanted with silicone devices. Even those not desiring the cosmetic use of silicone implants worried about the many occurrences of breast cancer, for they might one day be affected and later need reconstructive surgery. Some women who were not familiar with, or personally involved in, the silicone controversy considered the ban of the implants a government interference with their right to choose freely. They did not know just how dangerous these devices could be and what tragedy choosing them could inflict. Having suffered and survived the onslaught of silicone-induced disease, I knew.

In my opinion, measures to ensure our protection were years overdue. The FDA had promised that any eligible woman who experimented with silicone implantation would do so with a complete and accurate definition and explanation of all risks. Although grateful for the FDA's belated intervention, I realized upon closer examination that all was not as positive as I had initially perceived.

Though the advisory panel's provisions for women who wanted breast reconstruction after mastectomies seemed sympathetic, a number of breast cancer patients whose lives were already endangered felt that they were, as a result of their illnesses, "guinea pigs," chosen to be experimented upon. Many became angered by what they perceived as the FDA's inference that they were expendable.

For women implanted with silicone prostheses, the panel's advice offered no solution to their predicament, nor did they offer protection. In fact, they gave little in the way of reassurance. Their ruling seemed to present many contradictions. The panel warned of gel's leakage from implants and of the possibility of ruptures resulting from the deterioration of aging shells. The panel further prescribed the removal of an implant in the event of a rupture, presumably to circumvent the spread of silicone. At the same time, implanted women without signs of illness were advised not to remove their implants—a device capable of instantaneous rupture that contained, and routinely bled, a substance recently decreed unsafe. I felt, as did many others, some of whom were eminent authorities, that, at best, if the implant leaked only small amounts of silicone and women were "symptom-free," this was no guarantee against future illnesses.

In addressing the autoimmune illness issue, the panel had stated that it did not have enough data to conclusively prove a link between illness and the device. Panel Chairwoman Dr. Elizabeth Connell acknowledged that implanted women did report the development of the symptoms associated with autoimmune illnesses and assured them, "We are not ignoring it."[2] Nevertheless, the chairwoman cited a lack of determinate cause-effect data. The panel beseeched the FDA to conduct research study concerning the high incidence of autoimmune illnesses occurring among implanted women. Further, the panel implored the FDA to investigate the bleed and rupture rate of silicone-gel implants.

This request would not immediately provide the crucial information sought by millions of uninformed and questioning American women who had needed such information for many years. In what I consider an evasion of its responsibility to safeguard the public, the FDA had not instigated nor implemented a silicone implant study nor did many plastic surgeons insist on it. The manufacturers had also failed to conduct proper up-to-date testing.

# TORN ILLUSIONS

When scientific data does not exist, one may deny the occurrence of human illness.

During the February review, Dr. Norman Anderson stated that a 1993 FDA advisory panel had "literally begged" the American Society of Plastic and Reconstructive Surgeons (ASPRS) to organize a patient registry that would determine, beyond debate, the number of implant complications, injuries and illnesses. There had been agreement, Dr. Anderson said, "until the gavel hit the table."[3] Subsequently, the program was not enacted. Five years later, in 1988, another advisory panel chaired by Dr. Anderson again asked the ASPRS to form the patient registry. Dr. Gary Brody and the president of the surgeons' organization, who were both present at this FDA review, agreed to the panel's request. Dr. Anderson reported that, "within forty eight hours," Dr. Brody wrote a letter stating that the ASPRS had reversed its decision. Therefore, no registry was formed. If breast implants were as safe as many surgeons asserted, why would the ASPRS not have embraced the opportunity to collect proof of it by conducting follow-up exams of their implant patients?

The surgeon's guild did little to promote other scientific inquiry about silicone implants as well. Dr. Brody testified before the FDA Review that the organization's solitary contribution to the question of silicone implant safety was the sponsorship of an assembly of experts who congregated in Santa Monica for "an entire day" of debate. It is my feeling, as I am sure it is the feeling of many, that the health of so many trusting patients merits more than one day of vacation and conversation in California. In reporting the results of the 1989 Santa Monica meeting, Dr. Brody stated, "The conclusions were that this may be a real disorder . . . it must occur in a tiny number of women . . . and at that date there was no test to predict who might be at risk."[4]

Although surgeons were unable to predetermine who might experience a severe illness such as mine and those of thousands of others, the implantations were not only performed, but were, in many cases, also encouraged. I take exception to this seeming lack of concern for what was reported to be the "tiny number of women" who are and will be damaged. The number of women who would be affected could not be established; however, even if there was only one, no life should be cast aside as expendable. When I asked Dr. Blais, during a recent conversation, for his estimate of the number of women at risk, he responded that "over the next twenty years" each and every implanted woman could be expected to showcase the aftermath of their silicone exposure.

As the consequence of much malingering by the FDA, the medical community and the industry, the claims of missing data have resulted in an inability to clarify all the risks of illness. Many women, therefore, remain improperly warned and informed. Perhaps another contributing factor to this confusion and misconception surrounding silicone risks may possibly have been a strong desire to quell public panic and subdue frightened women. This attitude was evident during the 1992 review when one doctor remarked, "I think one of the first things we have to do is not have the American women panic."[5] Indeed, although the agency presented every aspect of silicone implantation for the panel's review, a discussion of the FDA's early evidence of silicone's carcinogenesis was conspicuously absent.

Noting everything that had not been disclosed, I feel that perhaps a little "panic" was in order.

Though little was said about the human cancer issue in February, the agency's FDA Update, published in May, discussed the human silicone/cancer risk, stating: "The possibility cannot be ruled out."[6] The same FDA paper listed the warning symptoms of the autoimmune illnesses that now develop in silicone-contaminated women. I do not think many women had access to the publication.

In my opinion, the agency has a distinct obligation to dispense public health information. To hold back any data, under the guise of protecting women from emotional turmoil, seems to me a grave injustice, placing women at an extremely unfair disadvantage as they attempt to form their own conclusions about silicone implants, based on the few facts available.

I also wonder if attributing such lack of disclosure to protocol isn't horribly unfair.

On April 16th, Commissioner Kessler announced his ruling upholding the advisory panel's recommendations. Silicone implantation would be restricted to eligible women, all of whom would cooperate in scientific study and be "carefully monitored" for many years.[7] The Commissioner stated that "tightly controlled research studies will be set up to obtain more information on safety and effectiveness." Acknowledging the special need of breast cancer patients, he both suggested and reinforced a limitation of the silicone-gel implant's cosmetic use.

The FDA outlined the protocols governing three stages of permitted silicone-gel implantation, as well as proposed clinical study. Stage one would begin shortly and permitted urgent-need reconstructive surgery for mastectomy patients in the process of reconstruction and for those needing implant replacements due to medical necessity, such as a rupture. Stage two was to follow and included patients requiring reconstructive breast surgery arising from mastectomies, congenital deformities and breast injury. In keeping with the panel's directives, all women were to document the saline implant's undesirability as an alternative, sign consent forms and enroll in a patient registry. Stage three allowed for both reconstructive and augmentation surgery. The group of women would be comprised of a number necessary for research study and was estimated to be 2,000. To satisfy the stage three requirements, manufacturers had to provide "carefully controlled research studies" of each implant model they wished to market.[8] Although planned for the fall of 1992, the program did not begin as scheduled.

Susan Cruzan of the agency's press office told me during a January 1993 telephone conversation that stage three had incurred a delay, because the manufacturers did not complete the necessary research of these models. After having consistently failed in all attempts to submit adequate proof of safety data to the FDA, it just might be that this is a difficult, if not impossible, task to fulfill.

Mentor Corporation and McGhan Medical Corporation are the two manufacturers who were supposed to begin participation in the 1992 FDA's program of restricted silicone implantation. According to Ms. Cruzan, McGhan did not participate in the commencement of either stage one or two urgent-need reconstruction programs due to FDA violations that had to first be corrected.

According to a March 31, 1992 FDA letter, McGhan's violations at that time were listed as the "failure to review and evaluate physician submitted complaints," including "complaints involving injury or any hazard to patient safety," and the failure to report occurrences of "capsular contraction, leaks, tears, ruptures, deflations [and] medical complications."[9] Nonetheless, in October of that year, the agency allowed McGhan to distribute their stockpile of one implant model, Biodemensional, to cancer reconstruction patients who had a temporary McGhan tissue expander in place and whose physicians had determined that they could not have satisfactory reconstruction with any other implant.[10] (The tissue expander is a temporary, expandable saline implant used to stimulate tissue growth in mastectomy patients.)

When the stage three "prospective clinical investigations" do begin—if ever—they will, no doubt, be turned over to the manufacturers. I recently spoke to Susan Cruzan again concerning the program's later initiation, and she commented that the status of stage three was "unknown" for the time being. (See "global settlement" fund, Chapter IX.) Other safety studies pertaining to the chemical compounds released from the gel and shell, the implant's shell strength and the physical and chemical changes within the body are also to be obtained from the manufacturers. The FDA's decision to appoint the manufacturers as the providers of this information is, in my opinion, foolhardy at best.

Moreover, the FDA intends to work with these manufacturers in organizing a registry to pass on any "significant" new findings to implant patients. Taking into account all that has transpired in the past, I think it is unrealistic to rely upon the industry to now produce findings of any kind, significant or otherwise. I would be surprised to see an FDA-organized patient registry in the near, or even distant future.

I am certain much conclusive evidence of the long-term effects of silicone implantation in relationship to cancer and autoimmune illness will come from studies of women already implanted with silicone devices. One plan for an independent epidemiologic study to be conducted by the National Cancer Institute (NCI), a part of the

National Institute of Health, was under discussion at the time of the FDA-announced protocols, but, over one year later, the program had still not received government funding. If the NCI program is introduced, it will be carried out by the study of only breast augmentation patients; inappropriately, breast cancer patients will not be included in the research effort. In objection, Representative Henry Waxman, Chairman of the Subcommittee on Health and Environment, wrote an April 1992, letter to Dr. Bernadine Healy, then Director of NIH, urging the inclusion of cancer patients in the NIC studies. He informed Dr. Healy that fewer than one hundred breast cancer patients have ever been a source of study by the implant manufacturers.[11] Disregarding his plea, Director Healy replied, in a May 5, 1992 letter, that breast reconstruction patients would still be omitted from the NIC studies.

Other epidemiological studies are in progress at New York University and the University of Michigan. Test results are projected within three to five years. However, the disease latency estimates have now been expanded. They are from six to twenty-two years. Conclusions quickly determined, then, would be poorly formed and possibly incorrect. In addition, while reading the May 27, 1992 FDA *Update*, I found out, to my disbelief, that these studies have been sponsored by the manufacturers. I wonder if such studies can truly be construed as unbiased research? One publication "found a history of endorsements by seemingly independent experts who failed to mention that they were being paid by the manufacturers."[12]

Commissioner Kessler had pledged during the FDA review:

> I am acutely aware that many women who already have
> the devices in place are eager for reliable clinical
> information. The decision announced today will require
> studies ensuing that information will be gathered so we will
> learn, once and for all, how safe these devices are.[13]

I wonder how the public today can be asked to believe that manufacturers, and others involved in making profits from silicone, will conduct unbiased research and acknowledge and report evidence of implant-associated complications, illness and death, while many of them are embroiled breast implant liability lawsuits. Many will face financial difficulties or even bankruptcy if silicone devices are completely withdrawn.

Dow Corning, which does not currently produce silicone-gel implants, proclaimed during the February FDA review that the company would initiate a ten million dollar research fund to begin the "study" of silicone. It sounded good, but I wonder how we can expect unbiased future studies when Dow Corning has taken the brunt of breast implant liability litigation and is being sued as the silicone supplier of eight percent of all cases filed.

One "favorable" study surfaced in 1994, strategically released the day before the global settlement program's opt-out deadline date (Chapter IX). This research, conducted by the Mayo Clinic, reviewed the medical records of 749 implanted women and 1,498 women without implants in Olmsted County, Minnesota, over an eight year period. The results claimed not to have linked silicone breast implants to specific connective-tissue diseases. A news article reported that "only morning stiffness was significantly increased among women who had received implants."[14] One should note, however, the research project was funded in part by the Plastic Surgery Educational Foundation, as acknowledged by the medical journal publication of the Mayo study. According to the *Washington Post* article, plaintiff attorney Aaron M. Levine has further "produced documents showing that as much as $174,000 of the study funds could have come from implant manufacturers and medical organizations that had an interest in the outcome."

Dow Corning was asked whether or not it had actually contributed to the funding of the Mayo research, but the company would not either confirm or deny participation. The information was "not available."

In addition to this criticism, even the researchers themselves "concede the study population was too small to catch the incidence of rarer forms of disease linked to implants." The women studied and the control populations all came from one small area—Almstead county. The news report stated that, due to two million implantations, problems might occur in large numbers of women, but not be found unless "as many as 200,000 women" were followed for "at least ten years."

Dr. Sidney Wolf of the PCHRG, described the study as "incredibly misleading." He concluded that "to draw any comfort from [the study] is to engage in misleading or delusional thinking." He referred to other new studies (Chapter VIII), which have indicated that silicone gel causes "various complex effects upon the immune system." Dr. Wolfe also faulted the use of medical records as a guideline, because problems may be "underreported."

Meanwhile, Keith McKennon, Chairman of Dow Corning, stated in panel testimony that the company would proceed with its policy of securing protective orders from the courts.[15] Concurrently, in the future, the chairman vowed to release any information that the FDA might request. It is very difficult to know what to believe. I wonder if Dow Corning will be forthright in relinquishing corporate date, or if the company will hold back some information. I also wonder if the FDA will share privileged information with the public. Based on my past experiences and research, I am skeptical. It seems to me that the precedent of privacy and partiality, counterproductive to Commissioner Kessler's attempted reforms, has long been adopted. The Commissioner will have accomplished a terrific feat if he is able to move forward what has been a history of indifference to duty.

The FDA did not announce that breast implants had silica in them until 1988; yet this information had been provided in the manufacturers' patents and was on record for many years.[16] The presence of silica, which can produce both autoimmune illness and cancer, makes breast implant recipients susceptible to these same risks. A summary prepared by FDA scientists that year brought up the risks and warned that the inclusion of silica made possible the development of "silicosis and other serious medical conditions."[17] Women and physicians were not informed, nor did the agency order silicone implantations halted.

The polyurethane-coated breast implant exhibited was another problem. After taking no action on the TDA cancer risk associated with the polyurethane foam implant, the FDA chose the manufacturer of this implant (also involved in liability litigation) to conduct studies of the TDA-contaminated breast milk issue.[18] The manufacturer, first as Cooper Surgical and, later, as Surgitek, in 1987 and 1988 hired independent scientists and laboratories to conduct safety testing of their polyurethane implants. However, the company did not proceed with the testing when some results of these studies showed the product could be hazardous.[19] Dr. Steven Woodward of Veterans Administration Medical Hospital in Nashville discovered that the foam breaks down inside the body of rats at a rate of fifty percent within two to eight months. The dissolution of polyurethane releases the chemical TDA, which is linked to the causation of cancer and birth defects. Another researcher under contract, Dr. David Black of Vanderbilt University in Nashville, detected the presence of the TDA chemical in the milk of nursing mothers.

According to internal documents, the manufacturer Surgitek, a subsidiary of Bristol Myers-Squibb, terminated a 1978 study of dogs exposed to silicone while it was still in process. They destroyed the test animals, whose diseased organs revealed extensive silicone-induced illness. The company's president issued the directives, "Sacrifice dogs ASAP" and "No organs of dogs in freezer."[20] This information was obtained and reported by the Human Resources and Intergovernmental Relations Subcommittee of the House Committee on Government Operations during their investigation of the FDA's regulation of silicone breast implants.

One year following the FDA's restriction of silicone-gel implant use, the subcommittee stated that women continue to be "unprotected" and placed at risk from the devices.[21] Despite the FDA's commitment to monitor the "urgent need" reconstructive and medical replacement operations, it was reported that the agency had not tracked, followed or even totaled the number of silicone-gel implantations. When the subcommittee demanded this information, the investigators learned that approximately one-third of current implant patients did not have a signed consent form on file. The surgery permission form that has been presented to other prospective gel-implant patients for signature in its final version was a "watered down" translation of the FDA's original draft. Subsequent consent form amendments seemed directed toward appeasing the ASPRS's protests over the agency's proposed implant warnings. The subcommittee's scathing report stated:

> Despite the concerns about the dangers of silicone that were exposed by the internal Dow Corning memoranda in February, 1992 and increasing evidence of the risks of silicone implants in studies conducted by plastic surgeons and scientists in recent years, medical associations have continued to pressure the FDA to minimize dangers to potential patients in their informed consent forms.[22]

Further, the subcommittee reported that the executive director of the ASPRS had written a June 5, 1992 letter to Dr. Alan Andersen of the FDA, which set forth the society's "dissatisfaction" with the agency's drafted consent form.[23] The FDA capitulated and several ensuing adaptations were proposed.

Relating to the number of implant-associated injuries, the FDA's original consent form stated that "it is not known how many women have had problems." This, along with the following statement, "Manufacturers have not provided to FDA adequate scientific evidence" of implant safety, was later deleted from the form. The revised form reads "Breast implants have been used in nearly two million women for thirty years." The revision implies an assumption of implant safety based on the devices' history of use.

Concerning the treatment of capsular contracture, the FDA draft instructed that closed capsulotomy procedures "must not be performed." In the later form, this statement, too, was omitted. Today's consent form advises: "This technique is not recommended by the manufacturer, because it could result in several complications, such as breakage of the implant. However, your surgeon may feel this is the best method for correcting the firmness." The revised form does not remind patients that a rupture might occur during the process.

Few of the newer implant-associated cautions outlived the consent form cuts; the ones that did were weakened to the extent that I feel they were only partially accurate. According to the subcommittee report, the FDA intended to warn that breast implants could interfere with a woman's ability to breast feed. Instead, that recommendation was replaced with the ASPRS's statement that "many women have nursed their babies successfully." Any risks associated with "successful" breast feeding were reportedly not reviewed. The original FDA warning of implant-related birth defects received further modifications. The form now reads, "Preliminary animal studies show no evidence that birth defects are caused by breast implants." In my opinion, this is an inaccurate statement of the facts since there is no evidence that any such studies exist. Moreover, the scant scientific evidence that is in circulation supports the occurrence of implant-derived danger to the fetus (Chapter VIII).[24]

The rupture and gel loss warnings that were to be included in the consent form were diluted. For instance, the finalized form infers that ruptures are infrequent, despite the fact that in June of that year an FDA *Consumer Magazine* reported rupture rates as high as thirty-two percent. Also, the gel's migration in the event of a rupture was inaccurately described as "uncommon." The Congressional Report concluded that this statement "is not based on data."[25] In the first draft, the FDA rightly proposed to warn of the gel's migration "to other parts of the body."

In the revised format, however, the consent form states that in the event both the envelope and scar capsule are torn, the gel "can travel" and be "squeezed into" only "the breast tissue or into the muscle or fatty tissue next to the breast, abdominal wall, or arm." This statement does not take into account data compiled at the February 1992 FDA review. The truth of the matter is that the fibrous capsule will not contain gel in any situation, and all implants bleed gel, which will then migrate throughout the bodies of these patients. The ASPRS also suggested inserting the word "lesion" as a replacement for the word "cancer," and rephrasing the warnings of autoimmune and connective tissue illness with the less descriptive terminology, "rheumatic disorders."

I feel that the ASPRS's priorities do not reflect the best interests of all implant patients. However, many surgeons who belong to this organization today privately acknowledge, and possibly also fear, the repercussions of silicone breast implant use. Unfortunately, most are reluctant to publicly renounce or reject the doctrine of so powerful an organization. I cannot help but wonder at the FDA's mind-set when I think of the effect its inability to stand firm on matters of breast implant safety reforms has had on the lives of so many women. This inability resulted in a stamp of approval on a consent form that does not provide the best and most valid information available to prospective patients.

Additionally, the Congressional investigation determined that the FDA had not "carefully monitored," as mandated, the protocols governing a woman's implantation. The subcommittee stated that physicians could, thereby, loosely interpret and apply the FDA's requirement that a woman have a "severe breast deformity" in order to qualify for silicone-gel breast implantation. This is an area of contention, as surgeons associated with the ASPRS have earlier defined small breasts in their letters to the FDA as a "disease."[26]

During conversations with Dr. Blais, he stated to me that the ASPRS had also sought to have third party insurers classify small breasts as a "disease." Therefore, silicone implant surgery might become a non-elective surgical procedure in cases of breast disease (small breasts). Although this might be profitable for surgeons, defining small breasts as a malformation or malady is an affront to female dignity. The Congressional report also stated that the FDA did not require the implanting surgeons to supply any documentation to the agency substantiating the fact that reconstructive versus cosmetic operations were performed. The FDA asked surgeons to fill out a brief form, which would then be sent to the manufacturer. Since the FDA did not retain the form, the agency would not have a list of the implanting surgeons, much less know the number of implantations performed per surgeon.

I regard the FDA's revision of the guidelines established to protect women as a betrayal of the highest order. Representative Donald M. Payne, Chairman of the Subcommittee, concluded the following:

> This report shows that the fox is guarding the henhouse,
> and, as a result, women are not always given the
> information needed for informed consent. . . . When the
> FDA was under intense scrutiny from the Congress and the
> media, they were more careful about their regulatory

efforts. When attention was focused elsewhere, it was business as usual at the FDA.[27]

I am afraid it's also *politics* as usual; while many tidy up after the public whitewash, silicone-implanted women are left to cope with the plethora of problems that remain.

Of these many unsolved problems, two of the most critical involve silicone leakage and implant rupture. The advisory panel's warning that implants have a limited life span is a warning to be taken seriously. In the de Camera study, fifty-one silicone implants were removed from thirty-one women; results determined that twenty-seven of these were ruptured, seven were leaking, and only seventeen were intact. The study shows an incredible rupture rate of over fifty percent, which is much higher that the rates cited by either the manufacturers or the agency.

FDA representative David McGunagle reported these results at the February 1992 FDA review after a panel consultant requested the de Camera study data. Mr. McGunagle added, "Ruptures and leakage are not rare in this study. There is an increase in the number of ruptured implants after seven years. The cause of implant rupture is unknown."[28] Although a seven to ten year estimate is generally agreed upon as maximum implant durability, the FDA stated that early ruptures of unknown origin also occur after relatively short periods of implantation. Irrespectively, all implants will deteriorate with age. Dr. Pierre Blais cautioned the February advisory panel:

> These implants decay with time. They decay physio-chemically. They decay mechanically. They decay by fatigue . . . the shells, through repeated usage, even though nearly static, even in patients who are not very active, will fail in the same way as metal fatigues in many respects, to which decay, chemical decay, will be added.[29]

To complicate matters, it may be impossible to identify implant rupture or leakage, as mammograms and ultrasonic sonograms are often unsuccessful in making this diagnosis. A normal reading does not ensure that one's implant shell is intact, and "silent" ruptures are frequent. Dr. Judy Destouet, a radiologist at Washington University School of Medicine, has conducted studies of 350 implant patients. She testified before the advisory panel that "we cannot differentiate on physical examination most of the ruptures. . . . The other thing is, we cannot image the posterior aspect of the implant, no matter what we use, whether it's mammography or perhaps even with ultrasonography . . . so we're not going to find them all [leaks] with those two modalities."[30] Dr. Kathleen Harris of the University of Pittsburgh Medical School tends to rely on the results of sonography, but reported a case in which a leak went undetected despite this and other methods of scanning. She confirmed that ruptures and leaks "may be invisible by any method—mammography or sonography—so there may be many more leaks that we don't know exist."[31]

Some radiologists report a degree of success in isolating shell disruptions and silicone formations with an outdated x-ray method called Xeromammograms, although these emit a higher dose of radiation.[32] Xerox has a toll-free number to assist in locating these machines. CAT and MRI scanning processes are also being studied for their effectiveness in visualizing implant leakage and rupture. Radiologists at the University of Florida Health Service Center in Gainesville have reported making strides in the detection of silicone leakage with MRIs through the addition of a radiowave-receiving coil to the MRI scanning process.[33] No other MRI nor ultrasound scannings involve radiation exposure.

For women who choose to remove their silicone implants either as a safety precaution or due to existing complications and illness, other problems arise. Surgery for removing the implants is not commonly covered by a patient's health insurance policy; so the expense of this type of surgery presents difficulties for many women who have implants. Several manufacturers offered financial contribution towards the cost of the implants' removal by 1992, but any receipt of moneys was contingent on signing a waiver of all liability and damages. (See terms of the "global settlement" fund, Chapter IX.)

If one is able to afford the explant surgery, plastic surgeons willing to remove the devices are difficult to find. During the 1992 FDA review, Dr. Harry Tobin, representing the American Academy of Cosmetic Surgery, attested to surgeons' reluctance to perform this surgery. He complained that "they are confused as to how best to advise [sic] their patients who are demanding to have implants removed . . . Many feel it is safer to refuse to treat former patients on the theory that they are protected by the statute of limitations."[34] Nancy Dubler, an advisory panel consultant, was offended by this statement and described the practice of patient refusal as "quite shocking."[35] Vivian Snyder, the panel's consumer representative, "was horrified" to learn that physicians would refuse to treat women after having placed implants in them.[36]

Dr. Norman Cole, former president of ASPRS, stated that if a physician "failed in his responsibility" to care for a patient, the ASPRS "will tend to take over that responsibility."[37] Although it is somewhat difficult to discern what his nebulous promise means, it is hoped that the ASPRS can be depended upon to assist implant patients in need of surgery. However, many women report that, although their physicians have not outright refused, some doctors have tried to deter women from removing their implants and have made them feel foolish for having either concerns or symptoms. A malpractice insurer, supplies their plastic surgeon subscribers with a specific consent form for removal surgery that has its own mode of discouragement. It warns of "severe psychological effects," including "depression," and the "loss of interest in sexual relations for such women and their partners."[38] It is no small wonder that women who previously were not informed of the most fundamental cautions relating to silicone implantation are now outraged. (One implant patient testified before the February review that "not once in twenty years was I ever told that the implant could leak, bleed, rupture or disintegrate."[39]) Surgeons remained silent, never expressing concerns over the mental health of their patients, during the booming years of breast implementation, while still reaping the monetary benefits of this type of surgery.

According to a support organization's recent newsletter, however, plastic surgeons are now proposing that psychological testing of all patients prior to both implant and explant surgery become a mandatory requirement.[40] (To register an objection to this proposal, see note 40.) Some surgeons have asked the FDA that they be designated the ones to conduct the proposed profile testing. In my opinion, not only are the surgeons unqualified to administer and decipher the testing, but the results might be judged with bias. In addition, the possibility exists that a surgeon's subjective interpretation of the test results could be used as a weapon against the patient if future implant-related litigation should arise.

I personally feel that it would be wiser for surgeons to come forward in support of implant patients, for, in doing so, liability lawsuits might decrease. I did not involve my own treating physicians in legal action because I do not believe that they knew about the dangers when information concerning silicone implants was not publicly available. I received implants during the early years when manufacturers did not reveal the research on these devices.

Later, as "newly available" information began pointing to the risks of silicone implantation, many surgeons either remained uninformed of, or overlooked, these risks. Today, however, physicians cannot afford to overlook the increasingly available scientific and medical data, or to be excused if they neglect to consider the implant as a possible cause of a woman's illness. I do not suggest that the majority of plastic surgeons are not giving priority to their patients' well-being, for it is known that many are. As a result, early diagnosis and the prostheses' removal may prevent medical disasters such as implant leakage and rupture. Additionally, those patients who wish to chance leaving their implants in place must be given a detailed explanation of any and all associated risks, as well as be informed that as their implants age, their chances of problems increase.

National and local support groups are helpful in providing the names of surgeons who perform frequent explant surgery (Appendix). Once acquainted with silicone illness, these surgeons find confirming evidence of this disease in both their observations and clinical studies.

Dr. Marguerite Barnett, a member of the ASPRS from Venice, Florida, is another surgeon who has performed well over one hundred explantations. Having identified the occurrence of silicone implant-associated disease in her patients; she said that the patients who come to her for explant surgery are motivated by "illness, not fear."[41] Dr. Barnett has reported a high recovery rate among her explant patients. She confirms that most of her patients' symptoms are alleviated, and that the majority of women improve after their explantation. When requested, Dr. Barnett replaces the silicone gel-fill implants with those containing a saline fill, but also performs the microvascular free-flap reconstructive procedures.

As my investigations continued, I spoke with many women who have had implants and were either uncertain what to do or had made up their minds to have them removed. They told me of both supportive and non-supportive surgeons. There are surgeons who readily acknowledge the risks associated with silicone-gel implantation and there are surgeons who are still in denial. Many advise their patients to replace their old silicone-gel implants with saline prostheses in order to avert eventual ruptures and gel migration. One woman, who was acutely ill, had a surgeon who refused to remove the ruptured implants because she could not afford the cost of the surgery. She was told to save her money for a year and return if she could then afford the surgery. I recommend in a case such as this that the woman contact an attorney who will make arrangements for the implants' removal.

At the time of the FDA silicone implant review, women who looked for guidance and advise from physicians other than their plastic surgeons discovered that medical professionals experienced with silicone-related illnesses were a rarity. So bewildered was the American Medical Association by the panel's recommendations that the society did not issue a statement. When Jama Kim Russano, founder of CATS (Children Afflicted by Toxic Substances) testified before the advisory panel, she echoed the sentiments of the many ill and frustrated women who can not locate medical treatment. Mrs. Russano stated that she has "personally spoken to hundreds of women with similar symptoms" who would have participated in studies had they been contacted. "I am appalled also," she said, "at the lack of education within the medical community. GYNs [gynecologists] not having information and telling women that they can breast feed their babies; top cancer doctors not knowing what a rupture or leak is."[41] She was further concerned that the FDA had not put forth a program of education for the physicians with whom women consult daily.

Due to the scarcity of medical information and physician expertise relating to silicone illness, women must often travel great distances to a few large medical centers that are equipped to evaluate and treat implant-related disorders. The National Institute of Health has only recently begun to study implant patients who have received diagnoses of autoimmune illness. Rheumatologists see the majority of women with these diseases although allergists and immunologists are also becoming well informed and knowledgeable.

Because of the current interest in silicone illness, Dr. Finegold presented a research study in November of 1993 of fifty-one patients experiencing silicone-associated disease to the American College of Allergy and Immunology at the society's annual meeting held in Atlanta, Georgia. Dr. Finegold and Dr. Vasey of the University of South Florida conducted a workshop together on silicone illness in conjunction with this meeting. (National and local support groups can provide referrals to other physicians who have experience with silicone disease.)

Since the ban of silicone implants, there are other indications of expanding awareness within the medical community. Most physicians who do treat implant patients conclude that illness is, indeed, resulting from silicone implantation.

A February 1993 *Wall Street Journal* article discussed "the growing number of medical researchers" who have linked the silicone-gel implant to "never-before-seen diseases of the immune system."[43] In confirmation of the medical testimony given before the 1992 FDA panel review, the researchers reported that the diseases "mimic the traditional diseases known generally as autoimmune illnesses," but exhibit different symptoms and laboratory results. "The disease is a disease unto itself," said Dr. Gary Solomon, associate director of the rheumatic disease department at New York Hospital's Joint Diseases Orthopaedic Institute. Although previously "skeptical" of silicone-associated illness before seeing implant patients, Dr. Solomon is now "convinced" of its existence. He reported that his patients have a "constellation of laboratory findings" that are not associated with any known illness.

# TORN ILLUSIONS

The same *Wall Street Journal* article stated that other physicians at Baylor College of Medicine in Houston reported on an implant patient who "developed badly disfiguring scleroderma" following an implant rupture "precisely where the escaping silicone had flowed." In contrast to the results of a recent Mayo Clinic study, Dr. Alan J. Bridges, a rheumatologist and associate professor of medicine at the University of Wisconsin, acknowledged, "Even people who were skeptical are saying there's just too much scleroderma" in implant patients. Dr. Bridges is following the medical history of 150 implant patients with immunologic abnormalities that deviate from the classic connective-tissue diseases. Dr. Lori Love, an FDA researcher who has studied the development of myositis (a very rare autoimmune illness) after silicone implantation, also reported symptoms and antibody findings that differ from those of traditional myositis. Dr. Eric Gershwin, Chief of Rheumatology and Allergy at the University of California accurately concluded that "reasonable people are not asking whether silicone causes disease, but how often." As more and more reports come out on silicone-caused diseases, plastic surgeons who once denied the possibility of serious illness resulting from implants have now begun filing lawsuits against Dow Corning for marketing an unsafe product that proved injurious to their patients.[44]

While implant dangers hover and threaten, women who search for a safe breast prosthesis learn that it may be years before new products are available. Manufacturers are in the process of researching substitutions for the silicone-gel implant and estimate that new breast implant prostheses will be formulated within three to ten years. One silicone-gel replacement under evaluation at the University of Washington School of Medicine in St. Louis is peanut oil—a natural substance that can be metabolized by the body without difficulty. Another alternative, a soybean oil fill manufactured by Lipomatrix, is encased in a "hard" silicone shell. The company "believes" that implant-associated problems are confined to a "particular" kind of silicone (a smaller molecular strain), yet whether or not the new device will "irritate" the immune system is unknown. Lipomatrix officials "concede there is evidence that silicone does provoke an immune response—at least in some people."[45]

For the time being, the invention of a safe implant shell devoid of immune stimulants continues to be sought. Hopefully, the silicone-gel implant experience will serve as incentive for manufacturers to carefully research, produce and market a safe, dependable implant prosthesis and take care to protect rather than endanger women's health.

At the moment, two choices are available for reconstructive or augmentation purposes. There is a natural alternative, which is known as the flap procedure. It requires a long and delicate surgical operation performed under general anesthetic. Tissue, fat and muscle are "tunneled" from other parts of the body (usually from the stomach or the back, and sometimes from the thighs) to the chest area for use in the formation of a new breast. The flap procedure is not suitable for all women; for instance, those who are very thin, those who smoke or those with diabetes.

The only prosthetic alternative is the saline (salt water) filled breast implant. This implant was only used in ten percent of cases before the ban on silicone-gel implants. Now, the number has doubled. However, it is often not as cosmetically successful as silicone implants. Saline implants may create an unnatural, rippled appearance of the skin, and their rupture can result in a sudden deflation of the device. A saline leak or rupture releases and distributes harmless salt water, unlike silicone implants where there is the possibility of silicone-gel loss and migration. However, saline breast implants are not without other risks similar to those of silicone-gel implants. The saline solution is contained within the same silicone-elastomer shell, and rheumatologists report the similar occurrence of complications and illnesses from saline implants. If one reacts to silicone, it is conceivable that even a small amount of the substance will provoke a reaction.

Moreover, the unrestricted saline implant has not been subjected to an FDA safety review. Although planned for the fall of 1992, the agency did not announce the proposal requiring saline implant manufacturers to submit their required pre-market approval (PMA) applications until January 5, 1993. This is possibly the beginning of a contest that will be just as drawn out and convoluted as the silicone-gel implant review.

During a January 1993 conversation with Dr. Alan Andersen of the FDA, I was given no explanation for the postponement of the saline implant review, which is now tentatively scheduled for 1995. I further questioned Dr. Andersen about the unrestricted use of two other silicone implants: the male penile and testicular prostheses. He replied that these medical devices, along with others containing silicone, were slated to have eventual FDA reviews in the order of their "priority." (Two other solid silicone implants used for male chest and calf muscle enlargement are also in use, but there are as yet no plans to review them).

As of March 10, 1993, the FDA reported it had received 5,948 MDR reports from manufacturers of injuries and illnesses resulting from saline implantation.[46] The agency did not state the number of saline implant-related illnesses that have been individually reported. Nevertheless, women should be advised that other toxic chemical compounds besides silicone are found in both the saline and silicone-gel implant shells. (The chemical additives that are found exclusively in the saline implant's are discussed in Chapter VIII.)

Implant risk, however, is not restricted to women. According to a recent *Sun-Sentinal* news article, approximately 300,000 men in the United States have had silicone penile prostheses implanted in them.[47] In a recent penile-implant lawsuit, the plaintiff contended that he had the silicone-implant related injuries of infection, disfigurement and immune system disorders. These problems are cited in many of the breast-implant liability cases. Some men have already received court verdicts against penile implant manufacturers, the largest manufacturer being American Medical Systems, Inc. of Minnesota. However, the current 1994 penile-implant legal action as stated by plaintiff attorney, Dan Bolten, "seeks to represent all buyers of such implants made by American Medical Systems" from the date the devices were first marketed in the 1970s.[48] However, there are many other medical devices using silicone. For instance, solid silicone implants for male chest and calf muscle enlargement are also in use.

# TORN ILLUSIONS

After learning that rheumatologists have reported the same autoimmune/connective-tissue disorders in silicone chin implant patients as in silicone-gel and saline breast implant patients, I decided to next research the other silicone medical devices currently being implanted.

# 8

## OTHER DEVICES,
## SAME DANGERS

I know now that our awareness of silicone problems has only begun.
Due to years of inaction by the FDA, silicone has found its way into
many unmonitored medical devices, none of which are without a
proportionate number of reported complications, illnesses and injuries
in association with their use or implantation.

Breast implants were the first silicone medical devices to
capture worldwide attention when thousands of escalating, associated
injuries and illnesses resulted from an exceptionally high implantation
rate. However, they are only the tip of the iceberg. Identical concerns
over the chemical makeup of silicone-gel implants and related immune
system disorders apply to all silicone-containing medical devices.
Panel consultant Dr. Thomas Krizek of the University of Chicago
asked Paula Wilkenson of the FDA during a discussion segment of the
February review whether or not D4, "the product that we're worried
about" in relationship to "immune phenomenon," could be
anticipated to come off his wrist implant and other implanted-silicone

devices. Ms. Wilkenson confirmed that D4 (Chapter VI) is an "inextricable, unavoidable component" of all silicone polymers. Dr. Krizek replied, "So what you have told me, then, is that this concern [FDA's] registered in your presentation regarding D4 and regarding immune phenomenon is something common to all implants—and not just to the gel implant, and would not exclude, for instance, say, the shell of a saline-filled implant?"

"Yes," Ms. Wilkenson replied.[1]

Silicone's medical use began in the 1950s when the ability of silicone oils to take on the characteristics of both a solid and liquid state attracted early interest from the medical community. Dow Corning responded with a Center for Aid to Medical Research in 1958. One of the first medical applications of silicone that originated from the Center's research was a silicone tube designed for the treatment of hydrocephalic children.

The past history of the utilization of silicone for medical use is equally fearful. Dow Corning had recognized the profitability of silicone's medical application and subsequently formed a Medical Products Division in the early 1960s. One primary medical venture produced a liquid form of silicone developed for cosmetic injection. The FDA classified the product as a drug and, thereby, gained regulatory control of its use.

In 1965, Dow Corning proceeded to apply for an FDA investigational exemption, for the purpose of conducting clinical experiments involving the same silicone injections. In this instance, silicone was to be injected for facial augmentation.[2] Nonetheless, at the time the company possessed reports stating that pure, unadulterated silicone had completely destroyed the breast anatomies of their laboratory animals. The FDA most surely was not aware of these findings. In response to Dow Corning's exemption request, seven prominent plastic surgeons secured FDA approval and permission to conduct clinical trials to correct facial defects using Dow Corning's silicone. The January 1992 moratorium banned this surviving practice.

The cosmetic treatment of human breasts with liquid silicone shots proved disastrous. After it caused serious illnesses and deaths,

Nevada and California banned the injections, as did the FDA. However, before the ban, the agency estimates that approximately 50,000 American women, most of whom were Nevada residents, received these cosmetic injections.[3]

Despite evidence showing silicone's destructive effect upon body tissue arising from the breast injection of silicone in both humans and animals, Dow Corning continued manufacturing and promoting it. Dow Corning seemed determined to develop silicone's medical market. In the next few years, company scientists invented many medical applications for silicone's human implantation; none have ever had their long-term biocompatibility "thoroughly established scientifically."[4]

According to Dr. Nir Kossovsky, a pathologist and medical implant expert at the University of California at Los Angeles, all medical implants are associated with a high rejection and complication rate. Blood clots, bone erosion, chronic inflammation, organ damage, systemic illness, connective tissue disease and even cancer may result from their placement within the human body.[5] "There is real cause for concern," said Dr. Kossovsky, for "the complication rate with implanted devices is frighteningly high." Although the gel form of silicone allows a greater degree of silicone migration, all silicon devices in both solid and semi-solid form shed particles of silicone.[6] The sloughing of these prostheses has been well confirmed by microscopic examination. In his book *Chemical Deceptions*, Dr. Marc Lappé further discusses the ability of solid silicone implants "to fragment and provoke mysterious systemic illnesses."[7]

The fragmented silicone particles have been shown to produce foreign body reaction in tissues surrounding urinary sphincteric implants, penile prostheses, temporal mandibular jaw (TMJ) implants, and hand-wrist implants.[8] Silicone granulomas have been found near the implants, and the development of lymphadenopathy and lymphadenitis have been reported.[9] Mayo Clinic orologists have identified silicone particles and foreign body granulomas in seventy-two percent of twenty-five patients with urinary and penile implants.[10] The majority of these implants were in place for less than two years. This study did not go so far as to establish the degree of silicone's migration via the circulatory and lymphatic system. However, Dr. Silver's 1993 medical literature publication (Chapter VI), which reported the migration of silicon particles to the sites of connective-tissue disease, offered numerous medical literature accounts of silicone's presence in adjacent lymph nodes. (This research related to connective-tissue diseases in association with silastic joint replacements.)[11]

Once silicone has reached the lymph nodes, distant migration becomes a distinct possibility. I found reports in my research that Synovitis has developed in patients exposed not only to silicone, but also to silica and silastic found in the protective sheath. Dr. Silver wrote that fractured silastic joint prostheses, which are composed of silicone elastomer, have been "well documented" to induce chronic inflammation of the synovial tissue in implant patients.

I found that reports of chronic inflammation with the development of Synovitis from silicone finger and joint implants began as early as 1974.[12] One study conducted by Dr. Peter Carter, attending hand surgeon at Baylor University Medical Center in Dallas, reviewed fifty-one patients with silicone carpal implants who were monitored for four years.[13] Osteolysis, which is a loss of bone, was detected adjacent to the carpal implants in fifty-five to seventy-five percent of those studied. Dr. Carter stated that many of these patients "were worse off than when we originally operated on them. They had more pain, less movement and they couldn't use their hand because it was weak."

Another study I came across involved thumb and wrist implants. It resulted in a 1986 publication by Dr. Clayton Peimer of the Hand Center of Western New York at Millard Fillmore Hospital in Buffalo.[14] He described eighteen patients who exhibited pain, swelling and bone destruction that developed within two to five years following implantation. As in the case of breast implants, removal of the prostheses relieved the patients' symptoms. He had notified Dow Corning with regard to his research in the mid-1980s, but the company did not respond. In 1991, Dr. Peimer reported seven cases of bone fractures occurring seven years after implantation. He contacted the FDA, who replied that they were "overburdened" with the breast implant issue, but "might" investigate the finger and joint implants at a later date.[15]

Despite the fact that many reports were sent to the agency, it wasn't until 1990 that a related FDA notice appeared in a Federal Register publication. It stated that "other silicone implants [in addition to breast implants] ... have been documented to produce sarcoma and other forms of carcinoma in humans."[16]  If I were one of those patients, I would feel as unprotected as a silicone breast implant victim.

How much "later" does the FDA intend to wait when questions of life and death are at stake? If corporations and physicians oppose surgical device reviews, as they did in the case of the silicone-gel breast implant, their views once again may not easily be opposed. The monetary gain for both manufacturers and surgeons encourages the continuing use of other silicone medical devices. Yet, because they have been used, it is estimated that ten percent of those with thumb and wrist implants will develop various types of hand or wrist impairment by fifty-five years of age.[17]

Silicone jaw implants, used for temporal mandibular joint (TMJ) disease surgery, are another device associated with many adverse reactions and complications. In 1985, oral surgeons at the University of Florida College of Dentistry at Gainesville, and the University of Texas Health Science Center at San Antonio, observed and reported immune responses in the parotid lymph nodes and surrounding tissue of eight temporal mandibular joint disease patients.[18]  They also reported incidents of inflammation resembling rheumatoid synovitis in tissue adjoining the jaw implant. Their medical paper concluded, "It is most probable that associated pathologic changes with a resulting dysfunction and morbidity may co-exist" with foreign body, granulomatous formations. The authors stated that "silicone may not be a totally inert material and its biochemical properties are not ideal for use in TMJ."

Problems with TMJ implants are an unceasing source of liability litigation. According to a recent *Wall Street Journal* article, many TMJ lawsuits are pending.[19]  One such legal action against Dow Corning was recently settled in Miami, Florida, and, according to the plaintiff attorney, the signing of a strict "gag" order was a prerequisite of the settlement agreement. (Chapter IX).[20] The negotiations were secret and out of court, however, the case and its subsequent settlement indicate that silicone injury, illness and death are not confined to a woman's breast implants. In addition, another 1993 TMJ lawsuit indicates that manufacturers other than Dow Corning are having similar problems. This lawsuit resulted in a $460,000 court award against Du Pont, the device's manufacturer.[21]

Other medical applications of silicone have also produced catastrophic results. For example, silicone has been used as an anti-foam agent in a device that oxygenates a patient's blood in cardiac by-pass surgery. In these cases, the silicone particles' entrance into the body blocked capillaries and resulted in tissue damage.[22] In a study of fourteen patients who underwent open-heart surgery aided by a bubble oxygenator, eight were found to have silicone droplets in their blood.[23] Five of the fourteen cases proved fatal; silicone was detected in the brains and kidneys of these patients.

As the same anti-foam agent, silicone has turned up in many drug products ingested daily. In one form, known as dimethicone, it is an ingredient in Di-Gel and other antacids. Infants are also routinely given derivatives of silicone, such as simethicone in non-prescription medicines to treat gas. However, an infant has unformed bowels and is more susceptible to digestive contaminants than adults. Although silicone remains in the digestive tract until excreted, the oral use of silicone has never been studied. Therefore, if adverse aftereffects did develop in the digestive tract, they could not possibly be recognized as being silicone-related conditions.

Diabetics, as well, are conceivably exposed to silicone during their day-to-day administration of insulin injections. Silicone is found in the piston of the syringe used by diabetics, and hypodermic needles are usually coated with silicone oil. It is important to note that diabetics frequently develop granulomas and inflammation at the sites of their injections, which partially explains why it is necessary for these patients to rotate among several different injection areas. It would be impossible at the present time, however, to differentiate between a silicone-induced systemic reaction in diabetics and the complications of the actual disease.

# TORN ILLUSIONS

Silicone tubing is another medical device associated with complications and disease. The use of silicone-polymer in the intubulation of nerves is reported to have produced injury to the nerve by eliciting a foreign body reaction that endangers neural function. The silicone tubing, which is impermeable to oxygen and nutrients, prevents nerve regeneration.[24] Incidents of silicone-induced endocaritis, an inflammation of the membrane lining the cavities of the heart, stemming from fragmented cardiac-pacing catheters inserted into the heart, have also been reported.[25]

In addition, there is evidence that the medical application of silicone tubing has caused many other serious, and at times deadly, complications. An article in one medical publication reported that some renal transplant patients, whose blood had been pumped through silicone tubing in hemodialysis treatment, developed liver scarring and various abnormalities. Silicone particles were found to be located in the livers of these patients. The author of that article stated, "This study confirms that silicone particles persist in the liver for some years . . . perhaps all patients who were/are dialyzed with silicone containing systems are at long term risk of liver damage." The diseases in patients developed within two to four years after the discontinuation of their hemodialysis treatments; other causes of illness of liver disease were ruled out.[26]

Other researchers reported a high incidence of liver disease having developed in kidney dialysis patients whose blood had been pumped through silicone tubing.[27] As early as 1981, there have been medical literature reports of mortal liver disease resulting from exposure to silicone tubing.[28] Following the deaths of some of these patients, pathologists, during autopsies, discovered a great amount of silicone particles in the patients' livers. This was later traced to the silicone tubing. Reports of liver disease and deaths stopped after non-silicone replacements were substituted for the silicone tubing. Although silicone tubing is still in use, Dr. Blais has told me that it now has a different formulation. I can only assume that all silicone tubing is made from this new formulation. It's hard to believe that manufacturers (by selling the product) and physicians (by utilizing their product) would further risk and sacrifice human life.

Presumably because of the enormous liability associated with the medical uses of silicone, Dow Corning has withdrawn from this endeavor. The company sold its medical devices business, Dow Corning Wright, in June 1993. The company continues to supply the small-joint silicone prostheses (Wright controls "eighty-five percent" of this market) until the new corporation, Wright Medical Technology, begins marketing its own orthopedic devices.[29]

However, silicone is silicone, regardless of its size, shape, form or supplier. We have reviewed some of the convincing evidence that silicone breast implants are not the only silicone product that causes serious illness, injury and death. We also know that men, as well as women, are harmed by these devices. These are the issues with which the United States and many other countries are finally dealing.

Worldwide action taken, in most instances, mirrors the FDA's restrictions in the United States.[30] Australia banned the use of silicone-gel devices in January 1992. Spain banned them and then formed a committee to study breast implant safety data. Italy extended an existing moratorium while collecting their own information. France's Ministry of Health recommended that physicians refrain from using silicone-gel prostheses until a panel studies implant safety data. Germany's Federal Health Office announced the same recommendation. In Ireland, surgeons voluntarily suspended cosmetic silicone-gel implantations. Although England did not limit the use of this breast implant, a 1992 publication in the highly reputed British medical journal *Lancet* reported a significantly high incidence of autoantibody findings in implant patients who exhibit silicone illness syndrome.[31] A study by Scripps Research Institute determined that women with implant-gel leakage displayed symptoms years earlier than women with intact prostheses.

At the time of the FDA Review in the United States, a confederation of eight European countries scheduled discussions on implant safety to be held in 1994.

However, many plastic surgeons in a multitude of nations abroad resent the restriction of silicone-gel implant use. Following the breast implant initiatives of the United States, surgeons from eleven European nations met in Amsterdam to sign a statement claiming that a ban was unwarranted due to a lack of scientific data to support it. In my opinion, a review of the 1,500 pages of FDA panel testimony proves otherwise. The fact that silica (asbestos), a lethal carcinogenic substance and immune system adjuvant, has been added to silicone breast implants (whether in the gel or shell) is enough evidence to ban further marketing of the device.

Almost two years after the FDA ban of silicone-gel implants, a commentary published in the *Journal of the American Medical Association* (JAMA) by Dr. David Kessler, Commissioner of the FDA, bolstered the agency's justification for maintaining the silicone-gel implant restrictions.[32] Dr. Kessler's paper came in response to the persistent urging of the American Medical Association (AMA), which moved to protect their physicians' rights to use the silicone devices.[33] Accepting the FDA's responsibility "for safety of products used in medical care," Dr. Kessler reprimanded physicians concerning their own responsibilities. The Commissioner referred to the thirty-year practice of implanting silicone prostheses in women "without having adequate information on what risks they might pose to their patients and without insisting on that information" as "an abrogation of responsibility."

Although Commissioner Kessler's "call for higher standards" may reflect the fact that he is "acutely aware" of the need to protect other women from harm, the countless silicone victims of today are the reminders of others' lack of concern in the past.

# 9

# A REVIEW
# OF SILICONE'S RISKS

Silicone, silica, chemical toxins, contaminants and compounds, most of which exhibit adjuvant and carcinogenic properties, are all present in breast implants and many other silicone-implanted medical devices. Although this chapter provides a factual evaluation of many hazards associated with silicone implantation, it is not my intention to cause undue panic, for the damage has already been done. Rather, I hope, the appraisal of these risks will serve to alert the public and their physicians to the possible illnesses arising from silicone implant exposure. Only with this information are implant recipients protected and able to safeguard their future health and legal rights. Of course, I regret not having this information available in 1980, when I had silicone implants, but today we have the data, and its message must not be ignored.

I understand, as well as anyone, that cosmetic surgery often achieves tremendous physical self-improvement. In many, it promotes an elevation of self-confidence and a positive self-image. When reconstructive surgery is necessary, the results may become a needed restorer of emotional health and well-being. Regrettably, in the case of silicone breast implants, these benefits are accompanied by calamitous health risks. To deny these risks and the frequency of their occurrence is a mistake. The body count of the silicone-injured and dead continues to spiral upwards, as research, testing, diagnosis and time advances.

The dangers are intrinsic to these types of breast implants: the silicone gel-fill encased in a silicone-elastomer envelope, the same gel-fill with a polyurethane-coated elastomer envelope, the saline fill also encased in the silicone-elastomer envelope and the double or triple lumen implant with a silicone gel-fill sack contained within one or two saline-filled elastomer envelopes. The reverse lumen implant has an interior sack encased in a silicone gel-fill elastomer envelope.

Any surgical operation entails the risk of developing complications. These include excessive bleeding, infection, adverse reactions to anesthetic and difficulty in wound healing. However, in addition to general surgical risk, there is now strong evidence that many other risks are serious and frequent. Further common complications that may occur within several months of breast implantation are a loss or increase in nipple sensitivity, persistent pain or discomfort, visible scarring and hardening of the breasts. Breast hardening because of capsular contracture occurs during the first six months after the operation in at least forty percent of patients, and can result in deformity of the breast.[1] Non-surgical treatment by external, closed-compression capsulotomy to break up the mass is no longer recommended, nor advisable. This procedure may precipitate an implant rupture.

Due to the occurrences, at different times, of capsular contracture, pain, implant rupture or silicone leakage, living with breast implants may, over a period of time, also necessitate repeated implant surgery. In addition, implant replacements offer no assurance that more complications will not develop. The number and kind of related complications as well as follow-up operations that any woman can experience may vary among each individual patient, but the likelihood of needing replacement surgery does not.

# TORN ILLUSIONS

The presentation of a 1988 study of ninety-seven patients who had implants removed, presented at the Symposium on Retrieval and Analysis of Surgical Implants and Biomaterials in Snowbird, Utah, reported "reoperation rates as high as forty-seven percent." The most frequent complications found were capsular contracture (at 71.3 percent) and implant ruptures with the bleed of silicone into the tissues (38%).[2] It is remarkable that all existing studies of removed implants indicate rupture rates that greatly exceed the FDA's own estimates. In a study of ninety-three explanted prostheses, Dr. Patten of Baylor College of Medicine in Houston, discovered an approximate sixty percent rupture rate.[3] Silicone implants have been described as "time bombs" ticking away in a woman's chest. It is a suitable analogy, as I have found out. We have learned that there is strong evidence all implants will rupture with time and age, regardless of a particular shell's integrity.

Ruptures cannot be prevented and many go unnoticed, although some are detected by a discharge from the nipple and a burning sensation in the chest area. These implant failures often cause gross breast disfigurement and have further resulted in women having to undergo partial and complete mastectomies with the removal of silicone-invaded chest muscles.[4] This possible outcome of silicone implantation should not be considered unexpected, as silicone has been shown to destroy the breast tissue of laboratory animals subjected to free silicone. However, this is not what a woman anticipates on the day she has breast implant surgery, and she is usually never informed that this complication occurs in others.

There is much evidence that silicone gel-fill implants allow the silicone to bleed through their outer shells. Even the double or triple lumen implant enables silicone gel to permeate the outer saline-filled envelope and enter body tissue. This occurrence is well documented in medical literature.[5] Therefore, women with lumen implants should not be overconfident that silicone leakage can be prevented in their cases. The alternative to silicone gel implants, a saline-fill implant, does not bleed silicone gel, but even these devices shed particles of silicone.[6] And even a modicum of silicone within the body may evoke reactions and migration.

The shedding of silicone from breast implant shells (as it sheds from any solid silicone prosthesis) is well documented, and the release of these silicone particles may even permit the deadly silica component to also escape from the outer shell. One cannot presume that the amounts of silicone and other toxic chemicals free to travel around the body are small and, thereby, of little consequence. Neither patient nor physician is able to determine the exact amount of silicone, silicon and silica the implant may be bleeding or shedding. The "minimal" amounts of silicone that all gel-filled implants continually bleed resulted in my own serious illness.

In the event of an actual rupture, massive amounts of silicone gain entrance into the body. This can result in devastating and protracted illness. A woman who has an implant rupture often suffers horrible complications, symptomatology and extended recovery periods.

Once it has migrated, silicone is irretrievable. In addition, we know that escaped silicone will readily travel via the lymphatic and circulatory systems, for it has been found in every organ and gland of the human body (Chapter IV). Silicone's permanent or indefinite presence in vital tissues of the body then offers unlimited possibilities for the development of disease. In constant stimulation by an "antigenic" adjuvant, the immune system becomes encumbered and overloaded while continuously combating a substance that cannot be metabolized, destroyed or entirely excreted.

Dr. Marc Lappé, renowned toxicologist and author, considers the very inertness of silicone to constitute the basis for this "paradoxical toxicity." In his book *Chemical Deception*, Dr. Lappé writes, "It is now evident that silicone and silica materials can stimulate the immune system to go after body constituents that are normally isolated from immunologic assault." Due to the chemical's stability and the inability of the body to remove the silicone, it "remains as a chronic source of immune stimulation, probably both because of the complexities it forms with normal protein components of the blood and tissue, and because of its adjuvant-like property."[7] This scenario will lead to the development of autoimmune/connective-tissue diseases and disorders. The incidences of related illness having occurred in women with implants flourish. As of June 1994, the FDA received from manufacturers 74,336 reports of silicone implant-associated illnesses, injuries and 52 related deaths, which are not inclusive of the reports filed by physicians.[8]

All implant patients studied exhibit distinctive and atypical clinical and laboratory findings that separate their diseases from any autoimmune/connective-tissue disorder known today. Significantly, as many as three-fourths of these women have abnormal immunoglobulins or autoantibodies that deviate from the traditional patterns of established illnesses.[9] One example of the deviance of silicone disease from others relates to the development of Sjogren's Syndrome, which is often diagnosed in women who have silicone breast implants. In the natural form of the disorder, lymphocytes are detected in the salivary glands; however, Dr. Frank Vasey has found that the salivary glands of some implant patients contain macrophages instead.[10]

A 1993 editorial authored by Dr. Vasey and his colleagues cited other reported abnormalities among some implant patients, which have now been recorded in current medical papers. Dr. Vasey stated that breast implant recipients experiencing dermatomyositis, a condition symptomized by purple rashes on the forehead and shoulders among other places, have a "high prevalence of human leukocyte antigen (HLA-DQAI*0102) compared with women with natural disease and control subjects."[11]

In a number of women with implants who develop Lupus erythematosus, antibodies to small nucleoproteins (sn RNP) have also been identified, although the patients lack other diagnostic indications of Lupus.[12] With regard to its application, Dr. Vasey writes, "This may indicate that immune stimulation occurs in women with breast implants and ill-defined connective-tissue disease." Antibody binding to a large molecular-weight protein is another abnormality identified in the serum samples of "seventy percent of women who developed rheumatic disease compared with less than five percent of patients with systemic Lupus erythematosus or rheumatoid arthritis and zero percent in the control subjects."[13] These findings are extremely relevant. While the majority of implant patients exhibit this atypical disease and unusual symptomatology, the same group display an imposing conformity of similar characteristics and symptoms of this atypical syndrome.

That same year, FDA's *Talk Paper* shed light on the silicone-associated autoimmune/connective-tissue illnesses that are increasingly being diagnosed in implant patients.[14] The paper discussed new immunologic research studies of silicon-gel, which will appear in a future journal publication.[15] The agency paper stated the following:

> Two recent animal studies have shown that silicone gel of the type used in breast implants can act as an adjuvant—that is, it can enhance the ability of the animals' immune systems to produce antibodies to an antigen (a substance that stimulates the body to produce antibodies).

That silicone could be an adjuvant was determined by injecting rats with a blend of cow's blood protein (which represented the antigen) and liquid silicone. The *Talk Paper* reported the following:

> Under these test conditions, the antigen [cow blood protein] alone would not have been expected to produce an immune response. In the presence of silicone gel or another adjuvant, however, it produced a strong antibody response.

The same FDA paper acknowledged the long-held concern that "silicone gel might provoke an immune response" in implanted women. The report concluded that "that is one of the reasons the agency decided to restrict the availability of these devices. These new studies are consistent with this concern." The research is also very "consistent" with the emergence of today's silicone illness.

This important information was not made immediately public despite the agency having promised, a year earlier, to circulate any "significant new findings" to implant patients. When the FDA distributed a breast-implant consumer pamphlet to those who requested related information, these animal studies received cursory notice. The consumer pamphlet referred to "recent animal research," that "reinforced the idea that there might be a link between silicone gel and effects on the immune system," without describing this particular study.[16]

The same FDA paper made vague references to "another study" which "has shown that some women with breast implants produced antibodies against their own collagen (a connective tissue protein)." The research referred to, which was conducted at the University of California at Davis, determined that one out of three patients studied had very "high levels of antibodies to key proteins in collagen." In fact, some of their antibody elevations were "unbelievably high."[17]

Breast implant patients and their physicians should have a detailed, timely report of any current data, especially such strong evidence of connective-tissue involvement. Despite the fact that I have been trying to accumulate all available evidence for many years, I still marvel at all that remains unknown and that which I am still discovering. For instance, until recently, I did not learn of one manufacturer's animal study, which exposed one hundred mice to heated silicone fumes. Each subject subsequently died from this exposure.[18] What has become increasingly clear is that a combination of self-reactive autoimmune conditions and chronic inflammation (aided by the surplus of chemical toxins provided by the breast implant) may initiate severe, systemic consequences in silicone-implanted women.

Doctors have observed, and researchers have seen, evidence of chronic inflammation and foreign body reaction in association with silicone migration throughout the bodies of implant patients.[19] Their studies reflect the findings of previous animal testing. Similarly, the development of silicone granulomas and lymphadenopathy, which often become painful and require removal, is frequently reported in implanted women. One 1989 FDA document had acknowledged the medical literature accounts of the silicone-associated inflammatory reactions and stated the following: "In humans, numerous reports described silicone granulomas or lymphadenopathy in distant organs such as axillary lymph nodes, liver, kidney and even the brain which demonstrate silicone migration in patients that underwent silicone migration five to twenty years earlier."[20]

The 1992 FDA advisory panel had voiced another inflammatory-related concern with respect to the capability of cytokines (the immune cells secreted by the inflammatory granulomas) to cause symptoms of illness in many implanted women. A cause-effect relationship has now received verification. Recent medical research has provided dramatic evidence of silicone's link to the development of cytokine-associated illness in implant patients.

According to a 1993 news release, cooperating researchers at several medical centers have conducted in-depth studies of chronic fatigue syndrome. This mysterious flu-like illness, which lasts for an extended period of time, results in debilitating exhaustion. Severe chronic fatigue symptoms are frequently experienced by implant patients; neurologist Dr. Bernard Patten reports of the condition in ninety-two of one hundred women studied.[21]

The three million dollars devoted to chronic fatigue research was financed by the National Institute of Infectious Diseases of Bethesda, Maryland. The study results determined that injections of cytokines into healthy volunteers stimulate the body to produce symptoms of chronic fatigue syndrome.[22] This research finding may also be supported by the study of chronic fatigue patients. When I discussed this discovery with Dr. Finegold, he remarked that he has noted an elevation of the cytokine (IL2) levels in some of his own patients who suffer this syndrome.

In reference to cytokine research, Dr. Stephen Straus, Chief of the Medical Virology Center at the National Institute, explained that chronic fatigue has remained "a profound mystery," as physicians have been unable to determine "the molecular basis for fatigue in anyone, much less in a person with chronic fatigue." However, the news article reporting the cytokine findings stated that researchers today "are now convinced" that the illness is authentic. "One compelling reason" is the new cytokine research; chronic fatigue syndrome is now believed to be caused by the abnormally produced cytokines.[23]

The chronic fatigue symptoms of implant patients, therefore, might have originated from silicone-associated foreign body inflammation. A theory put forth during the February 1992 panel review by panel consultant Dr. John Sergent, Chief of Medicine at St. Thomas Hospital in Nashville, added another dimension to the cytokine breakthrough. Dr. Sergent stated, "One of the hypotheses about scleroderma" is that it "may not be an autoimmune disease, but a disease in which the primary problem is a production of fibroblasts and endothelial perforation induced by cytokines; for example, in response to some environmental toxin."[24]

A research paper supplying concrete evidence of the silicone/cytokine link was presented at the annual meeting of the 1993 American College of Rheumatologists. This paper reported findings of "large amounts if IL-2" (cytokines) in the breast biopsies of implant capsules removed from patients.[25] In the past, during the course of litigation, some manufacturers have often attributed an implant patient's ills to the "imaginary" and unrelated chronic fatigue syndrome. Today, this claim has been proven false.

The migration of silicone further evokes extensive organ and gland damage in implanted women, with ensuing tissue necrosis, just as it has in test animals. Tissue damage in the diseased organs and glands removed from implant patients is reported to be associated with the presence of silicone. Whether by chronic inflammation, immunologic reaction, or chemical aggravation, multi-organ failure involving the lungs, kidneys and liver has occurred in implant patients.[26] At times, it even proves fatal. These organs—including the skin and immune system—are responsible in large part for the body's defense against foreign and toxic invaders. In the process, they may be the ones most adversely affected.

The human brain is another organ where silicone has been shown to migrate. Not surprisingly, therefore, silicone-associated central nervous system involvement and dysfunction continues to be reported. Dr. Patten's Baylor group currently follows over 3,600 implant patients who exhibit these disorders. Abnormal brain scans have been determined in twenty-five to thirty percent of one hundred Baylor patients, with short term memory loss occurring in seventy-eight of one hundred women studied.[27] Nerve biopsies showed abnormalities and damage in seventy-nine percent of the patients, and seventy-two percent experienced loss of pin prick sensation in the lower extremities. Of the numerous abnormalities that are detected in silicone implanted women, however, none fit into any diagnostic category of any known neurological disease.

One medical literature publication provided additional evidence of silicone's ability not only to insinuate itself into the nervous system, but also to cause neurological disease. This particular research determined that silicone's infiltration of a peripheral nerve resulted in constricting neuropathy following an implant rupture.[28] I feel the detection of a silicone-invaded, diseased nerve holds serious implications of neurological involvement in implanted women, as well as limitless possibilities for the development of associated illness. The neurological illness that is currently reported, which reflects possibly both a self-reactive immune response and chemical neurotoxicity, should not be taken lightly.

Later this year, Dr. Patten and his associates documented another implant patient's death, supplying more evidence that fatalities as a consequence of this aspect of implant-associated illness (in conjunction with multi-organ failure) do, in fact, occur.[29] Circulatory system complications, blood clots and vascular diseases, which are as potentially life-threatening, can also develop. At least one death from a fatal stroke was reported in a woman under thirty years of age. After all other causes had been ruled out, her death was attributed to the migration of silicone.[30]

Women exposed to silicone with resulting illness and medical complications generally become susceptible to chronic and recurring infections. This may involve a damaged immune system, cytokine activity or even the discovery that breast implants may be a breeding ground for many dangerous microorganisms.[31] These microorganisms have been found both inside and outside the prostheses, in body tissue and thriving in the shell's glue.

In studies of implants retrieved, Dr. Blais reports the presence of organisms "never before found in the human body." The microorganisms that are isolated from breast implants fall into these categories: fungi, water borne bacteria, microbacteria, sulfate metabolizing bacteria, anaerobic bacteria and pseudomonas. The latter pathogen, pseudomonas, is associated with lethal hospital-contracted infections capable of causing death. The contamination of breast implants by a wide range of microorganisms may be a result of improper and inadequate sterilization. The manufacturers, nevertheless, distributed the implants as "ready to use" and rarely, if ever, did the surgeon perform other implant-sterilization procedures.

Although Dr. Blais has discovered "thousands of growing, living organisms" in all of the various types of breast implants removed, he finds the saline implant to be more at risk of contamination than the gel-filled prostheses. Its valve, which is necessary for the intraoperative filling of the saline solution, provides easy access for the microorganisms to both enter and exit. To make matters worse for saline-implant patients, surgeons who are responsible for formulating the implant's sterile, saline-fill solution frequently include additional ingredients. Dr. Blais refers to the ensuing saline mixtures as "cocktails" to which cortisone, antibiotics, antiseptics and even psychotropic drugs were added.[32] (Silicone-gel implants were also treated with locally applied chemicals for the same purpose.[33])

According to Dr. Blais, the psychotropic drugs (which are mood-elevating antidepressants) and other additives were included in the saline solutions as an experiment to reduce or eliminate capsular contracture. The experiment was not a success. However, one might ask if it displayed a degree of disregard on the part of many physicians for their patients' health. Unbeknownst to the patients, the doctoring of the saline fill exposed many saline implant patients to possible serious chemical reactions and interactions. Even today, many of these patients continue to assume that their implants contain only a sterile saline/water solution.

A chronic or simmering infection through implant contamination places added stress on a recipient's already compromised immune system. While an implant patient's health can steadily deteriorate due to one or more of the numerous silicone-associated diseases and complications, there is the possibility that further stress caused by infection can result in the collapse of the entire immune system. Dr. Finegold supports this theory with the following illustration.

He explains that cytokine activity (part of an immune response) occurs when a virus or substance such as silicone becomes deeply embedded in the genetic make-up of cells, thereby inciting prolonged inflammation, as occurs in chronic fatigue patients.

Many of these patients are afflicted with chronic viral infections and subsequently develop an acquired-immune deficiency as a result of their inflammatory illness. The ultimate breakdown in the immune system of implanted women may also be a forerunner to cancer, long reported in both animals and humans in association with silicone implants. For example, an aggressive form of lymphoma (defined as immunoblastic sarcoma of B cells) is related to preexisting immunologic disorders or an immuno-suppressed state.

Just as it has been for me, the cancer risk associated with breast implants is a primary concern of all silicone-implanted women. In order to evaluate the cancer connection, it is necessary to assess the evidence implicating the implant as a contributor to the disease.

Even if, for discussion's sake, I accept the idea that implants themselves do not actually cause cancer, the fact is that all breast prostheses interfere with the early detection of breast cancer.[34] This risk factor is equally shared by all silicone-implanted women and occurs in spite of the two-view mammography screening recommended for implant patients by the FDA. During the special screening, women with breast implants require twice the number of pictures than do women without prostheses. This doubles the amount of radiation exposure which women with breast implants must receive to obtain films. Nonetheless, these films do not image the entire breast. Mammograms are not usually recommended for women under thirty years of age; nevertheless, young women who have implants need earlier and more frequent mammographies (including the required two-view screening), because these women are most susceptible to breast radiation-induced cancer. The degree of mammography-associated radiation exposure may be minimal, but the effects are increased in implanted women and should be reviewed.

A 1990 study conducted by Los Angeles cancer specialist Dr. Melvin T. Silverstein had reported that silicone implants concealed approximately forty percent of all breast cancers in implanted women (a forty-one percent false-negative rate) despite the two-view mammography screening.[35] In an earlier study conducted in 1988, Dr.

Silverstein determined that only sixty-seven percent of cancerous tumors were diagnosed. These are somber statistics. In view of this, one certainly does not need to tempt fate by extensively or permanently exposing one's body to chemicals exhibiting carcinogenic properties.

According to the 1992 FDA panel testimony, both the gel-filled breast implants and even the less obstructive saline implants are known to obscure up to eighty percent of the breast tissue in some cases. The estimates may vary, but generally at least half of the breast remains hidden from cancer detection efforts. As a result, small tumors often go undetected.

One implant patient who developed breast cancer following augmentation mammaplasty testified before the 1992 FDA review, telling the panel that two mammograms performed separately by reliable radiologists within ten days of a breast biopsy failed to discover her advanced tumor. This late diagnosis resulted in her doctor's prognosis that she had a fifty percent chance of living for five years. Her story graphically depicts the reality of risk with regard to delayed cancer diagnosis.

Dr. Susan Love, a breast surgeon and author of *Dr. Love's Breast Book*, stated that one out of every thirty women may expect the occurrence of breast cancer.[36] With a family history of the disease, the odds increase to six out of thirty. There are several calculations used in determining the cancer risk. The above figures represent the relative risk; another calculation factors the probability of a woman developing breast cancer by age seventy-five. These figures state that approximately one out of every twelve white women and approximately one out of every fourteen black women will get the disease.

With regard to a silicone implant patient's risk, the FDA has estimated that ten percent of the women implanted with the prostheses will develop breast cancer.[37] This projected figure is higher than Dr. Love's relative and probable percentage of disease risk affecting the general population. The inevitability that one out of every ten women who elect to place a breast implant within their body will then develop a cancer, which may not be diagnosed, must be considered an unacceptable risk by anyone's standards.

The silicone implant's ability to influence the course of breast cancer results in serious and lethal complications. Early detection of breast cancer can prevent the loss of a breast. Regardless of size, retaining a natural breast is always preferable to losing one, and certainly a temporary increase in breast size is not worth losing one's life.

The later a malignancy is discovered, the greater the danger. Furthermore, medical research has reported that women who develop breast cancer following implantation have a higher incidence of invasive lesions and involvement of auxiliary nodes with more positive lymph node findings.[38] This complication indicates that, when cancer develops after breast implant surgery, there can be a rapid spread of the disease to other areas. Such a possibility adds another dubious and gloomy aspect to the prospect for recovery. The discovery of further spreading cancer is particularly awful for a mastectomy patient who has undergone silicone implantation.

The fact that breast cancer shows more activity and aggression in women who have silicone breast implants than in those without them may suggest something other than that their struggling immune system is under assault. It might also signal that breast implants can cause the actual development of the disease.

In researching the silicone implant as a causative agent, several aspects of breast implantation must be explored. A prime consideration is that, upon placing a foreign object permanently within the body, there is an inability to predict what a woman's own genetic predispositions and individual reactions may be. Moreover, any implanted foreign body can stimulate, induce or hasten the development of cancer (Chapter IV). Foreign body cancer is not, as some manufacturers have purported, "solely a rodent phenomena." Reportedly, it has occurred in all species of mammals—including humans.

It is also important to remember that any implant shell, regardless of its particular fill, contains threatening chemical components and catalysts (substances sometimes used to activate and achieve desired chemical reactions). Many of these activators and other included chemicals are proven carcinogenic agents (Chapter VI). Examples are silica, or asbestos, which "when administered. . . . produces a sarcoma at the site."[39] Whether as an additive or by-product, silica is found in all breast implants.

The chemical catalysts used in the manufacturing of breast implants are, themselves, sources of special concern. One such catalyst is dichlorobenzoyl peroxide.[40] At the end of its chemical reaction, the benzoyl peroxide cleaves in two. Although one half joins part of the silicone molecule, the other half becomes hostile and free to move about. Benzoyl peroxide is not only deemed an irritant, but is also a foreign oxidizing agent. Oxidation, defined as a loss of electrons, occurs with a removal of molecules (or electrons) that are necessary for normal oxidation functioning.

Benzoyl peroxide causes abnormal oxidation throughout the body. (I believe this process was, to some extent, involved in my peculiar chemical and metabolic reactions to my silicone implants. Some physicians suggested that an "abnormal" oxidation problem was occurring in my case). Chloroplatinic acid is another catalytic agent added to silicone oil as the precursor of the gel.[41] Although chloroplatinic acid, in its original state, had anti-tumorigenic properties and may be used in cancer chemotherapy, in the case of the silicone-gel chemical process, the acid reacts with molecules to form cis-platinum, a recognized carcinogen and a chemical able to modify proteins and cause DNA changes.

Silicone gel is home to many complex chemical substances, including cyclics (substances which remain in the gel after the completion of the chemical process as a by-product), which are pharmacologically active. So active, according to Dr. Blais, that these cyclics were proposed for medical use by Dow Corning as psychotropic drugs, earlier defined as tranquilizers and anti-depressants. Dr. Blais also stated that corporate documents certify the fact that Dow Corning patented several of the cyclics contained in implants.

The presence of cyclics in silicone gel is more than unsettling, for one can imagine possibilities for chemically-induced neurotoxicity and even an alteration of the psyche in women who have implants. Moreover, Dr. Blais has reported that the cyclics are capable of derailing calcium metabolism, which results in an aggressive depletion of bone mass. I am now experiencing this bone density loss. Whether it is due to the premature loss of my silicone-invaded ovaries and my consequent estrogen intolerance, or the acceleration of the process by the calcium-robbing cyclics, this condition resulted from my silicone implants.

The public has now been further informed that many of the chemical components of both the implant shell and the silicone gel-fill remain unknown. In questioning what the ingredients really are, as well as their indeterminate effects upon the body, we find that the chemicals already named are capable of promoting disease and death. This is not a new discovery. Dr. Lappé writes that, by the 1930s, "no one would dream of intentionally putting raw silica into the human body, because silica dust had been shown to cause acute illness and death or a chronic lung-damaging disease known as silicosis when the dust was breathed. When inhaled into the body, its effects last almost indefinitely."[42]

In spite of silica's infamous history, Dow Corning included this substance in their devices. I believe other manufacturers may have made equally poor choices, and could have included other pernicious chemical toxins in their devices.

Women whose implants are or were coated with polyurethane have increased carcinogenic exposure, as the breakdown of the foam inside the body releases the chemical TDA, which is known to produce liver cancer in laboratory animals. The presence of TDA has been detected in the breast milk, urine and recently in the blood of patients implanted with polyurethane-coated implant devices.[43] To date, these prostheses are also associated with the development of human malignancies at the site of implantation.[44]

The dangers of polyurethane are well-established and well known. In fact, many manufacturers have required their industrial workers to wear breathing apparatus and protective clothing in the workplace to prevent occupational exposure to this substance.[45] Strangely enough, while carefully protecting the people who were working to produce the polyurethane, the industry distributed thousands upon thousands of these polyurethane implants to be placed inside the bodies of women.

Dr. Blais, a veteran of the Canadian Health and Welfare Bureau of Radiation and Medical Devices, was instrumental in exposing the polyurethane-implant risk. He discovered that the foam was originally developed for industrial use, such as the upholstering of furniture. From his research and investigation, Dr. Blais learned of the polyurethane foam's tendency to break up once it is placed within the body. From 1986 through 1988, he had written repeated memorandums to other bureau officials regarding the dissolution of the implant's foam covering. By 1989, Dr. Blais had publicly declared the implant "unfit for human implantation." Later, both the FDA and the Canadian Health and Welfare Bureau confirmed incidences of internal breakdown of the polyurethane, with subsequent releases of TDA into the body.

Although the implant was voluntarily withdrawn from the United States market in 1991 following this public disclosure, Surgitek continued to sell the product to women abroad. As a matter of fact, when Dr. Britta Ostermeyer-Shoaib of Baylor Medical Facility returned from a 1993 trip overseas, she reported to me that fifty percent of European breast implantations are still performed with polyurethane implants. A December 1992 court case in the United States involving the polyurethane prostheses became the first implant liability case to reach court following the 1992 FDA moratorium. The trial resulted in a twenty five million dollar award against Bristol Meyers-Squibb, Surgitex's parent company.[46] Perhaps they will now rethink the decision to distribute their polyurethane implants overseas.

In order to assess the ramifications of breast implant additives, it is relevant that carcinogens are able to retain their capacity for producing biologic reactions at very low dose exposures. The perilous breast implant provides a notably prolonged exposure to these agents whatever their amount. Dr. Lappé has stated that most malignancies can be "traced to a single cell of origin."[47]

In my opinion, any discussion of silicone implants' potential for causing cancer must include an evaluation of the indications and evidence that silicone is, itself, a carcinogen. Concerns that silicone might be a carcinogen date back to the 1950s, when breast injections of liquid silicone were believed to be directly related to the development of malignant tumors. Early animal studies lend support to this belief. "Silicone and other polymers," including polyurethane, were found to induce up to a fifty percent incidence of cancer, "predominately sarcoma," in rodents at the site of the polymer's invasion.[48] Dow Corning's rat studies, conducted from 1985 through 1987, which used a dose amount comparable to the human dose exposure, also produced findings of a "pronounced" increase in the occurrence of sarcoma in the rodents. The same results were obtained from the two silicone gels tested.

Dow made no public announcements about this very significant finding, nor another important prior Dow study. In the earlier study, no tumor increase was detected in the same strain of rat after exposure to the solid outer-envelope membrane.[49] The results of the newer test strongly suggest that silicone tumorigenesis is not only a foreign body phenomenon.

Although "solid state" foreign body tumors are invasive, they do not usually metastasize (spread via the blood stream). The Dow Corning two-year rat study, however, reported a high incidence of metastasized sarcoma throughout the bodies of the laboratory animals.[50] Evidence of the spread of malignancy was found in the animals' hearts, lungs, stomachs, pancreases, kidneys, livers, adrenals, skin and thymus. In addition, "the gel implant associated malignant tumors ... were found only in the treated rats."[51]

In the company's earlier 1968 studies, widespread lymphoma was found in silicone-exposed mice. This increases the probability that the resultant tumors cannot be attributed to the solid state or physical form alone, but instead to the chemical characteristics of silicone. Taking all into account, it is clear that the combination of so many known cancer factors, incorporating foreign body-induced cancer, carcinogenic additives and silicone as an indicated carcinogen, can only result in dire silicone implant/cancer consequences.

The long period of latency associated with the development of chemical-related cancer further hinders the accurate evaluation and

estimation of future repercussions. Underscoring the important latency aspect of the disease, tumor occurrence in silicone-exposed rats is estimated at two-thirds of a lifetime. The following examples, as adapted by the Public Citizens Health Research Group from the 13th International Cancer Conference in 1982, illuminates the human latency factors:

chromium—lung cancer—20-25 years

radium—bone sarcoma—23 years, low dose

35 years, high dose

vinyl chloride—liver angiosarcoma—21 years

aromatic amides—bladder cancer—14-45 years

nickel—ung cancer—24 years

asbestos—lung cancer—30 years

asbestos—esothelioma—37 years

When we consider that silicone implantations have been performed for only a little over twenty years, it is obvious that the optimal time to have cancer studies is still years away in most cases. Proper epidemiological studies, which require a follow-up of fifteen to twenty years at the very least, have never been conducted or begun. Dr. Lappé has stated that studies of "thirty or more years" are typically needed "to observe fully the effects of exposure to carcinogens." Having knowledge of the data to date, I would not elect to participate in a premature experiment like the controversial Deapen Study, nor wager on the ultimate results.

The Deapen Study, conducted by plastic surgeons and epidemiologists who were hired by an implant manufacturer, followed 3,111 implant patients for an average of only 6.2 years.[52] The study, which reported no higher incidence of breast cancer in women who have silicone breast implants, seems to me clearly flawed and incomplete. The majority of the women (82%) included in the research were less than forty years old. Having such a short follow-up

period, plus choosing women of such young ages, highlights the shortcomings of this study.

In criticism, the FDA stated, "This study has not contributed greatly to our understanding of the relationship between breast implants and breast cancer."[53] A discussion paper of the Deapen Study, authored by Dr. Lynn Rosenberg of Boston University School of Medicine in Brookline, Massachusetts, also faulted the study, due to its inadequate follow-up of patients. She stated, "This is important, since it is well known that many years can elapse between the occurrence of an exposure and the occurrence of a cancer."[54]

Despite its shortcomings, what the Deapen Study did determine and report was an alarming increase in the incidence of cancer found in other areas away from the site of implantation. Regarding this determination, the FDA stated, "Based on these results, and the fact that silicone can migrate to other sites, the authors should have addressed this issue by including examinations of cancer at other sites, instead of limiting the study to only breast cancer." Dr. Rosenberg's paper, as well, noted the increase in the development of tumors distant from the implant site. Her paper concluded: "Finally, it is of concern that the observed number of cancers at sites other than the breast among the women who had undergone augmentation mammaplasty was fifty percent greater than that expected, and this result almost reached statistical significance."

In light of the earlier mentioned evidence that established the occurrence of metastasized, malignant cancer in animal studies (polyurethane-coated implants have also been associated with tumors found in areas other than the breast in laboratory animals[55]), the Deapen Study findings concerning human beings are disconcerting, to say the least.

An evaluation of the breast implant/cancer association involving remote tumors is complicated by the amount of time it takes to develop a cancerous tumor, as well as the time factor for silicone's lengthy travel via the lymphatic and circulatory systems to organs and glands targeted for disease. For these reasons, many tumors that turn up years later, located far from the implant site, might not be

# TORN ILLUSIONS

accurately attributed to the actual source of their origin—the silicone implant.

Nevertheless, the evidence in human beings that these tumors are silicone-associated (whether through silicone migration or cancer metastasis) is convincing, for it corresponds with findings in animal studies. Silicone which has migrated has been found coexisting not only in the cancerous breast tissue of implant patients, but also in removed cancerous, lymphatic, uterine and ovarian tissues.[56] Again, this bodes ill for implant patients in the future.

The simultaneous finds of cancer and migrated silicone in female reproductive organs is also an ominous sign for women with silicone implants. Moreover, the involvement of sensitive reproductive organs and their complex hormonal processes happens more frequently than was supposed.

Silicone which has migrated is often detected in the reproductive organs of women with silicone implants. In my own illness, the presence of migrated silicone resulted in a chronic inflammation severe enough to necessitate the removal of the glands. Like me, other women have lost their ovaries, and many have undergone hysterectomies due to silicone-associated disease. Sybil Goldrich, founder of Command Trust Network, is one example. In her case, silicone was found to have migrated to the liver.[57] When the disheartening post-implantation complications necessitate hysterectomies and ovariectomies in young women of child bearing age, they are rendered incapable of conceiving children.

Although silicone does appear to have somewhat of an affinity for inhabiting our reproductive organs, the physical presence of silicone in the ovary or uterus is not needed in order to experience dysregulation of the ovarian-produced hormones. Irrespective of silicone's location in the body, it is known to attract and absorb the ovarian hormones (both estrogen and progesterone) as readily as it does the body's lipids.[58] The knowledge of this capability dates back to the early 1960s. Referred to as the Judah Folkman effect, the discovery resulted in silicone's use as a coating for the IUD (intrauterine birth control device).

This ability of silicone to both absorb and store female hormones may also be evidenced in my history of silicone reactions. Without having ever exhibited menopausal symptoms or taken estrogen replacement therapy, I was still found to have abnormally elevated estrogen levels five years after the removal of my ovaries. At the same time, the testing of my serum showed elevated FSH levels and an undetectable progesterone level indicating a lack of ovarian function. (These tests are used as a standard measure of ovarian function in women.)

Dr. Finegold then discussed my curious hormonal situation with Dr. Norman Anderson of Johns Hopkins School of Medicine. Dr. Anderson was the first physician to attribute my abnormal estrogen levels to the silicone/hormone-absorbing phenomenon. Although the adrenal gland may, in some instances, produce small amounts of estrogen, even my gynecologist considered my estrogen levels too high for too long a period of time to be explained by anything other than silicone's storage of my own estrogen (previously produced by my ovaries before their removal).

Dr. Pierre Blais, with whom Dr. Finegold also conferred, agreed with this explanation and predicted that my silicone-stored hormonal surplus would eventually be depleted. He was correct. My estrogen levels, which were being monitored, did subsequently decrease. It was apparent at this time, due to my age and my premature loss of hormonal function, that there was no remaining or functioning ovarian tissue. Therefore, ovarian tissue had not contributed, nor could it explain, the prior five-year high elevation of my estrogen levels after my ovaries were removed.

A question now being asked by researchers and others concerns the effects of excessive amounts of abnormal silicone-stored hormonal concentrations in women who have silicone implants. One of the prime concerns involves the female hormone/cancer connection. The body's hormones carry out their functions at very low levels of concentration. Therefore, it follows that the possible uptake of female hormones by silicone, resulting in high levels at the implant site, may be a cause of increased incidence of breast cancer, as had occurred in the animal studies.

## TORN ILLUSIONS

The body's hormones must maintain a state of delicate chemical balance. Dr. Lappé writes that "disturbing this exquisite balance can lead to disease. . . . When hormonal levels are disturbed, a cascade of physiological reactions commonly ensues."[59] Some of the "most important" are those reactions involving cell division, because protracted hormonal stimulation may result in cancer. Carcinogens derive much of their potency from their interaction with other molecules, especially the hormone molecule.

Dr. Lappé presented the following example: In some animals, only females develop cancer after exposure to a carcinogenic substance. Female rats, for instance, develop liver cancer when injected with dioxin, yet males do not.[60] Significantly, when the rat's ovaries are removed, the dioxin/cancer effect is eliminated. It is interesting to note that Dow Corning frequenly used male rats for silicone testing.[61] Thus, the company did not record an increased cancer inducement in the possibly higher-at-risk females.

The same cancer/hormonal relationship exists in human beings. Breast cancer risk increases with the overall number of years in one's lifetime that ovulation has occurred.[62] So crucial is the hormonal/cancer link that if the ovaries are removed at an early age without estrogen therapy, the cancer risk is known to be measurably reduced, reflecting the estrogen's cell stimulating effect.[63] While one level of cell stimulation may be necessary, it can be harmful in abundance. Consequently, high levels of estrogen and progesterone have long been associated with the development of cancer in women, as evidenced in the history of the drug diethylstilbestrol (DES) and birth control pills.

The original testing of the prototype of the birth control pill began in 1957 using six to nine times the hormonal dose of today's pills. The dose amount was halved two years later, but still exceeded three to four times the current dosage. In the 1970s, when high dose estrogen pills were in use, related liver adenomas or carcinomas were found in women after treatment with the drug.[64] Before using the pills, none were at special risk of developing liver disease and tumors (all of the same type). These exhibited characteristics never before, in medical history, recounted. Many questioned whether the tumors could have been avoided if scientists and physicians had learned the lesson of the DES catastrophe.

In animal testing conducted during the early 1940s, DES, a synthetic estrogen later used to treat miscarriages, produced growth stimulation, accelerated breast cancer and abnormal reproduction in laboratory animals. The reliability of the animal study findings are borne out in today's first and second generation DES victims. Although some of the mothers developed DES-related breast cancer, some of the daughters, who received exposure to the drug years earlier in the womb, developed both reproductive abnormalities and cancer.

One of these second generation reproductive problems involved adenosis, which is an abnormal accumulation of tissue near the cervix; another was the abnormal development and deformity of the uterus. A rare form of vaginal cancer next appeared in the DES-exposed daughters. These occurrences were attributed to the use of estrogen in a synthetic form until 1979 at which time researchers discovered that the administration of naturally occurring hormones could elicit similar pathological changes.[65]

Rats treated with "normal" estrogen also developed the same adenosis-like tissue growths, with a sudden "unnatural burst" of natural estrogenic compounds. These, when given "at the wrong time," can disrupt the normal uterine development and cell production in newborn rats.[66] (Newborn rats were chosen for treatment because their organ development is equivalent to that of a human fetus in the late stages of pregnancy.)

The significance of these studies is not easily missed; one may logically conclude that silicone is delivering the same "unnatural burst" of stored estrogenic compounds in profuse amounts at equally inappropriate times. Accordingly, the possibility for an increase in the cancer risk, as well as fetal development abnormalities from silicone-related hormonal repercussion, is adequately supported and well within the realm of scientific probability.

One illustration establishes not only silicone/hormonal interplay, but also the need for concern. It has been reported and documented that a percentage of implant patients who are treated with birth control pills begin lactation (the production of breast milk).[67]   The solitary medical explanation for this is silicone's involvement in the hormonal process. (This does not occur in women without breast implants.) The bizarre occurrence of lactation suggests silicone-induced dysfunction of both the ovaries and the pituitary; for lactation does not begin without pituitary stimulation and the breast having first been "primed" by estrogen.

In the case of breast milk occurring in implanted women, estrogen provided by the birth control pill has either been misdirected or misused. Additionally, breast leakage (but not actual lactation) is routinely experienced in silicone-implanted women who are not treated with birth control pills. Although this occurrence has often been reported, as yet research has not been conducted in this area. Unfortunately, with such strong indications of silicone's serious interference in the normal hormonal functioning of human beings, one can hardly suppose that either mothers with silicone implants or their children will escape the consequences of implantation unscathed.

Another problem is teratogenicity, a toxic substance's ability to cause embryo/fetal death, retarded growth and other structural as well as functional abnormalities in the womb. Questions are now being raised concerning breast implant-associated fetotoxicity, but fetal susceptibility to chemical agents has already been proven. The fetus is known to be very accessible and greatly at risk to very small amounts of toxic substances during the first trimester of pregnancy.[68]   The vulnerable fetus is often harmed by chemical agents that the mother may safely tolerate. Among the substances which do harm are alcohol, the antibiotic tetracycline, coumadins and heparin (anticoagulants), lithium (an antidepressant), toxidone (an anti-inflammatory agent), alkylating agents, cocaine, DES and the tranquilizer thalidomide.

In the late 1950s, thalidomide experiments resulted in both deformity and loss of limbs in the children of mothers to whom the drug was administered. Thalidomide was marketed mainly in England, Germany and Australia. By 1961, the majority of related birth defects were reported in these three countries. However, during this period, the thalidomide tragedy was not commonly known about elsewhere.

Due to this, the FDA, in 1960, permitted sixty investigators to conduct clinical testing of thalidomide while the agency processed the drug's approval for distribution in the United States. Upon learning of thalidomide-related deformities having developed in children overseas, the FDA swiftly canceled the manufacturer's application for a marketing permit. Soon afterwards, the agency discovered that the manufacturer, nevertheless, had already circulated the drug outside the clinical trials among 1,200 American physicians; the manufacturer did not inform these physicians of the thalidomide-associated birth defects that had occurred in Europe.[69] Of course, many preventable tragedies occurred.

Like thalidomide, silicone breast implants harbor an assortment of menacing chemical toxins and carcinogens. (This is particularly true in the case of the low molecular weight chemicals, one of which is silicone.) Many of the toxins and chemicals are able to pass from the mother to the fetus through the placenta, which is the organ that joins the mother and child and provides nourishment. For carcinogens that require activation, Dr. Lappé has written, "The placenta serves as a veritable chemical factory, with some of the richest enzyme-based systems for biotransforming chemical into active carcinogens ever found."[70]

Increasing concern, Dr. Lappé further stated that "agents that have high cancer producing ability are usually also potent gene-damaging agents (and vice-versa). . . . Specific genetic changes at identified locations on the chromosomes (including the sites for so-called onco-genes) are now well established."[71] One example is the chemical cis-platinum, found in silicone implants as both a carcinogen and teratogen. The chemical TDA, released from polyurethane-coated implants, is another carcinogen that has also produced birth defects in laboratory animals. These and many other toxic chemicals contained in breast implants can and do reach the fetus.

With regard to silicone, its low molecular weight enhances its ability to penetrate the placenta and enter the fetus. Once silicone reaches the fetus, its presence increases fetal endangerment, for silicone is an "oil" molecule. According to Dr. Lappé, fat (oil) soluble chemicals are known to be stored in fetal tissue, "especially in the brain."[72] The fetal storage of silicone can occur, then, in infants as it does in their mothers.

Researchers, physicians, and the FDA have been alerted to the information presented in this chapter for a very long time. Although the FDA has occasionally stated a concern, it has not inaugurated silicone implant/fetotoxicity study during the course of breast implant use. The agency's expressed (yet neglected) "concern," however, is perhaps derived from its own knowledge that silicone was proven to disrupt normal fetal development in rabbits when administered into the uterus and peritoneal cavity by injection.[73] These studies were originally conducted because silicones were intended for use in intrauterine devices (IUD).

Another troubling discovery has been obtained from one of the few fetotoxicity studies available. While a study conducted by Bates reported no teratogenic effects from silicone's injection along the spine of rats, other implant studies established a dose-response relationship to the development of fetotoxicity and skeletal abnormalities in rats and rabbits.[74] The higher the dose of silicone, the greater the effect, with rabbits showing the most significant results.

Many manufacturers appeared to have paid little attention to these problems despite the warnings that there could be dire consequences for future unborn children. Now, many women whose children were conceived after silicone was implanted in their breasts find that the results of future research will arrive too late. Evidence of second generation silicone-associated injury already exists; in addition, implant-associated miscarriages and stillbirths have been reported.[75]

I recently spoke to a woman from North Carolina who told me of having lost five sons through miscarriages following her implantation. Her physician had attributed these losses to "severe inflammation of the reproduction system." Reminiscent of the effects of DES, it has also been reported that several fetal-exposed children under the age of five have developed signs of early puberty.[76]

Illnesses among children of mothers who had silicone implants (second generation illness) are now occurring with symptomatology identical to that of the silicone-implanted mother. The uniqueness of the mothers' clinical and laboratory findings are being repeated in their children. Dr. Eric Gershwin, Chief of Rheumatology and Allergy at the University of California at Davis, is presently treating cases of second generation illness of children.[77]

He has concluded that these children are, indeed, at risk of developing implant-related disease. Dr. Gershwin described the illnesses he finds in these infants and children as "atypical autoimmune diseases," the same diagnosis given to the mothers. Dr. Gershwin fears that silicone "may cross into the breast milk and not turn up for a number of years. We've seen a number of children who've had a disease that we feel is possibly related to nursing with silicone implants."

The risk of breast milk contamination by silicone and other noxious chemicals is not an issue for all silicone-implanted mothers. Many experience an inability to breast feed after having breast implant surgery.[78] Several post-implantation complications are responsible for the loss of this function. Changes in nipple sensation is one such complication; an increase in nipple sensitivity will result in painful nursing attempts and may preclude breast feeding. In contrast, a decrease in nipple sensitivity also prevents successful nursing if the nerves involved in breast feeding do not signal the release of the breast milk. These nerves may be cut and permanently destroyed during an implantation surgery. Breast engorgement with the bursting of blood vessels is another complication that occurs in mothers who have had breast implants. Women whose implants are placed near the nipples develop the most difficulty in nursing.

I feel that other implanted women who have retained their nursing capabilities must become aware, for the wellbeing of their infants, of the possible risks associated with breast feeding. The possibility for second generation exposure to silicone and other harmful chemical toxins contained in the implant through breast milk contamination is should be a real concern. It has long been known that toxins are often transmitted from nursing mother to child via breast milk. For this reason, doctors strongly advise against the consumption of alcohol by nursing mothers. Regardless of the available medical knowledge concerning breast milk transmission of toxins, as well as silicone implant safety issues, the FDA has never addressed or evaluated the implant-related breast feeding risks. While the issue remained hushed, many implanted women nursed their babies.

Not only were these mothers not warned, but they were reassured about breast implant/breast feeding safety without there being any substantiating data to support this assurance. Pamphlets containing false claims of breast milk safety were circulated among implant patients; until 1991, the ASPRS was still distributing a patient brochure that erroneously stated, "Current studies suggest that you do not have to worry about silicone seeping into your milk glands." In fact, the so-called current studies did not exist. Moreover, Dr. Patten's Baylor group have reported finding the presence of silicone in the milk ducts of implant patients.[79] Once there, silicone's travel to the breast-fed infant is unencumbered. Silicone-induced illness could then develop in these children, just as it develops in their mothers.

A 1994 news article reported a recent development concerning breast implant/breast milk danger, as well as a direct link to silicone causation in the second generation illnesses found today. A publication in the *Journal of the American Medical Association* (JAMA) cited a new study of children who were breast-fed by mothers with silicone breast implants. The research determined that six of eight babies nursed by mothers with breast implants developed abnormalities and impairments of the esophagus.[80] The disorder, described as scleroderma-like (a term now very familiar among implanted women) did not affect the infants in the control studies or those who were bottle fed. This research must be considered the loudest alarm bell yet to sound regarding the threat of silicone exposure to the children of implanted women.

Unfortunately, silicone exposure is not the only threat. A breast-fed child is not spared harm from the plethora of additional chemical toxins, adjuvants and carcinogens that are present in silicone implants. One such chemical, TDA, has already been detected in breast milk. It stands to reason that any of the chemical contaminants released from the implant are capable of polluting the breast milk to the same degree. If any dangerous implant-associated microorganisms are present in the breast area, they, as well, might be transmitted to the breast milk. It is even possible that all implant toxins and poisons can be passed to the breast-fed child; to presume otherwise is foolhardy.

To advise a mother with breast implants to risk nursing her infant, years before unbiased research conclusively determines the complete consequence of breast milk exposure, is poor advice. The catch word here is "unbiased." I do not believe such research should be done by manufacturers of these devices.

In 1993, New York attorney Denise Dunleavy began the process of initiating and filing litigation (a class action lawsuit) as a means of providing medical monitoring for second generation victims. The purpose of the legal action was to obtain funding for research. (See Chapter X, terms of the "global settlement.") A detailed, related questionnaire has been distributed to women with breast implants; the Children Afflicted by Toxic Substances organization (CATS) assisted in organizing the inquiry (Appendix).

CATS was founded by Jama Kim Russano after her children developed illnesses secondary to her own silicone-associated disease. The organization has presented evidence before the National Institute of Health and the FDA. Medical experts in eight fields have also joined together to promote silicone/second generation illness research. Many other physicians watch and study the developing illnesses in these children.

Meanwhile, women should realize that tomorrow's research will, in large part, be obtained from today's experiments with children exposed to implant toxins both *in utero* and through breast milk. While the evidence and incidence of second generation illness grows, mothers, who have silicone implants and who have nursed children, become angered and distraught. To have incurred injury themselves is grievous enough, but to have damaged their children as a result of their implants is horrifying.

Many physicians conclude that the silicone illness of implant patients is "a disease unto itself." It is a specific, unprecedented syndrome embodying chronic inflammation, self-reactive autoimmune/connective tissue disease, neurological illness and toxic reaction. All of these merge into "never before seen" combinations of symptoms, clinical observations, laboratory findings, organ damage and immune dysregulation. Though it is considered an unknown disease, thousands of women experience the same symptoms.

One has only to attend a breast implant seminar, as I have, to be overwhelmed by the striking similarities in the illnesses about which these women speak. At least knowing they are not alone is of some support. I experienced silicone illness before learning that anyone else had ever contacted it. I was alone with a disease so horrible that I often thought I would die. Though the disease is no less horrible, now there is comfort in not being alone. One woman after another shares a similar story about themselves and their children.

My physician, Dr. Finegold, now describes the illness he encounters in implant patients as SAD, Silicone-Associated Disease. He told me that he thought of the name while reading the manuscript pages of my book.

As in my case, the disease begins insidiously; vague symptoms become bothersome in women like me who were healthy and active before implantation. As the symptoms intensify, new ones arrive. In the early stages, women often attribute their complaints to other factors. They begin to take vitamin supplements, lessen their work load and limit stress. Gradually, their health continues to worsen while the symptoms do not abate. In the event of a rupture or leakage, the onset of illness may be immediate and may rapidly accelerate.

The strange illness will develop and progress in the case of routine "bleed" from silicone gel-fill implants, just as it progresses in cases of silicone/saline-fill prostheses. Once begun, the illness will not halt; without fail, it will proceed. Eventually, a woman may become completely incapacitated, as I did, or worse, die.

There is no known antidote for silicone-associated disease, other than having the implants removed. Women, who have increasingly constitutional symptoms over a period of time or abnormal laboratory findings without an attributable diagnosis after comprehensive medical testing, should not delay in removing their prostheses. Many women report that their illnesses advanced at a slow, steady pace, then suddenly became critical. By this warning, I do not mean to alarm, but to forewarn, as the illness has proven to be lethal in some. I came very close to being one of them.

After consulting with physicians and scientists, I would further recommend that women consider the removal of the capsule surrounding the implant. Some surgeons advise leaving the scar capsule in place to hopefully achieve a better cosmetic effect; however, the capsules have been found to contain both silicone and chemical contaminants. I am grateful that Dr. Finegold had the wisdom and foresight, at a time when so little was known of implant risk, to order the removal of my own scar capsule.

Once those with silicone implants decide to have them removed, it is also important for these women to issue a stringent request that their implant or its remains be returned to them. An implant is a woman's property. Some women have gone into surgery with these instructions pinned on their hospital gowns. The implant or the remainder may be sent to Dr. Pierre Blais for testing (Appendix).

Once the implants are removed, many women's symptoms may dramatically disappear, possibly within days. However, complications from neurological, gland, or organ involvement may require more time. For some there often is a two or three month period before actual progress begins. For others it takes much longer. Yet, as I did, the majority of women do begin to recover. Most of the symptoms disappear as well, although this can be an extended process. Just as it takes weeks, months or even years, for symptoms to appear, it may take an equally long time for recovery to take place. My own course of illness over a period of years can be considered average. However, a woman may be more or less severely affected. Do not be discouraged. After having their implants removed, some implant patients who have been diagnosed with rare and unvarying autoimmune or neurological illnesses have made total recoveries without medication, treatment, or relapse.

This kind of recovery is one of the most remarkable and encouraging aspects of silicone implant-associated illness. It is now estimated that seventy percent of the systemic symptoms relent, and three-fourths of all women improve; many completely recover. I believe the number of recoveries will increase over time.

# TORN ILLUSIONS

Only recently have large numbers of women begun to remove their implants. Women who have breast implants of any type should carefully monitor themselves. Mild but persistent warning signs that intensify with time, as well as development of new symptoms which do not respond to medical treatments, indicate the possibility of implant-related complications.

Although many of the symptoms women with implants experience may appear to be general, it is not "normal" to have a majority of these symptoms, which continue to increase and worsen. If a woman develops or is experiencing such symptoms, a thorough immune system work-up by a qualified physician or laboratory is a necessity. Children born or nursed after women have implants must also be monitored; for these infants and children can exhibit the same symptoms the mother has.

Concerned women—those with the implants in place or already removed—may wish to have the ELISA (Enzyme Linked Immune System Antibodies) test conducted (Appendix). This is a blood serum test that detects the body's production of antibodies to silicone and one's sensitivity to the agent. Two doctors who conduct this screening are Dr. John Heggers and Dr. Nir Kossovsky. Immunosciences Laboratory also offers silicone antibody testing, as well as a complete immunological profile and a chemical antibody screening. Balco is another laboratory that conducts silicone serum study. This lab was cited by the esteemed British medical journal *Lancet* as one of the top laboratories in the United States.[81] For toxicologic testing, Dr. Hildegarde Sacarello-Staninger, a toxicologist who serves on the National Board of Directors for the Desert Storm Coalition, may be contacted. (Toxicology is the study of poisons, their actions, detection and treatment of conditions caused by them.) Dr. Sacarello-Staninger is familiar with silicone poisoning.

Removed implants can be sent to Dr. Pierre Blais, as mentioned earlier. Scanning processes may further aid in identifying silicone problems. MRI and SPEC scans determine brain inflammation and vascular problems; EEGS may show brain abnormalities; Gallium scans, which image soft tissue, visualize lymph nodes and locate areas of infection in the body.

In addition, women who have undergone a surgical procedure (not restricted to breast surgery) after their breast implantation—regardless of whether their implants have since been removed—should have their pathology tissue checked for the presence of migrated silicone. Tissue is routinely removed at the time of any surgery and stored in hospital pathology banks; tissue slides are available upon request. They should be sent to pathology researchers experienced in detecting the presence of silicone and resultant foreign body cell reactions. Dr. Nir Kossovsky and Dr. Douglas Shanklin are two pathologists listed in the Appendix who conduct this study. A word of caution: the identification of silicone in one's tissue may not be possible at local laboratories unaccustomed to this type of study, and its presence may be overlooked if not specifically sought.

There are many symptoms associated with silicone/breast implant illness. Though the list is long, each and all of these symptoms in variable degrees and combinations are often experienced and reported by implant patients:

1. Chronic headaches

2. Increasing fatigue

3. Increasing weakness

4. Breast, neck, shoulder and rib cage pain

5. Swollen lymph nodes

6. Acid-like burning sensation of the skin involving any part of the body

7. Swelling and/or redness of any part of the body

8. Breast leakage or discharge through the nipple

9. Hair loss

10. Unexplained rashes of any kind

11. Generalized itching

12. Loss of appetite, weight loss and nausea; colitis and bowel irritability

# TORN ILLUSIONS

13. Recurring fevers

14. Drenching night sweats and chills

15. Flu-like body aching

16. Ringing of the ears

17. Visual disturbances

18. Difficulty in breathing, shortness of breath

19. Any unexplained organ or gland enlargement and dysfunction

20. Unusual smell to urine

21. Skin thickening or tightening

22. Joint pain, swelling, redness

23. Morning stiffness

24. Generalized pain and weakness (fibromyalgia)

25. Raynaud's syndrome: sensitivity to heat and cold, swelling and redness of the fingers and hands

26. Sjogren's syndrome: dry eyes and mouth; in some implant patients, dry vagina

27. Muscle spasms and twitches that may progress to involuntary trembling, shaking and jerking of the body

28. Difficulty in swallowing

29. Generalized nerve pain

30. Short term memory loss

31. Loss of sensation, abnormal sensations (pins and needles, cold spots, tingling and numbness of the extremities)

32. Dizziness, lightheadedness

33. Loss of balance

34. Increasing hypersensitivity to previously tolerated environmental chemicals, medications and foods.

35. Unusual menstrual problems

In addition to the ones on the preceding list, other symptoms are found in children:

1. Mouth ulcers

2. Acid-like burning sensation in the mouth, throat and chest

3. Fingertip discoloration

4. Night sweats with a salty discharge

5. Recurrent stomach pain, especially after meals

6. Severe constipation

An astonishing aspect of silicone implantation comes to light in determining the number of women and children who are at risk of developing a silicone implant-related disease. At the present time, no test exists to predetermine those who may be susceptible, nor those who will succumb. So great is the possibility for physiological damage resulting from the development of the many associated illnesses that a woman's predisposition alone cannot be the basis for predicting the eventual occurrence of disease. Women become ill without having any prior individual or family history of the disease to which they fall prey. Exposure to silicone and a barrage of other toxins can be prolonged. The fact that there can be a long latency period is also critical in any chemical exposure. A woman's tolerance of the implant today does not provide security against tomorrow's disaster.

How many are at risk? Given time, truly all women with implants are. No woman is either exempt or immune, safe or protected from the consequences of implant use; neither are their children. How many women are already ill? No one knows, because for every silicone illness diagnosed, I fear others inevitably go undetected.

# 10

# THE VICTIMS:
# WHAT LIES AHEAD

The cryptic nature of silicone disease holds perplexities today and uncertainties in the future for those who are implant victims. The long passage from implantation to illness—culminating in diagnosis and a restoration of health—is painstakingly slow. Most women recover, but not all are able to withstand nor outlast silicone's rampage. Some have been permanently damaged in the process. Others will likely die. One implant patient with whom I spoke recently has received a diagnosis of progressive and fatal lung scarring, which physicians attribute to her silicone exposure. She represents only one of many who will probably become silicone fatalities.

Although I consider myself one of the more fortunate silicone victims, I have endured unbearable pain during my fight for survival. I well recall having told several of my doctors during the early years of illness that I did not believe it possible to feel so ill yet remain alive.

As I well know, the suffering caused by the disease is not restricted to physical trauma. This illness invades every aspect of the

# TORN ILLUSIONS

victims' lives. Social and economic hardships are heavy burdens. With poor and declining health, victims withdraw from activities and functions they enjoyed prior to their implantations. Finding themselves becoming progressively confined, as I once did, a great number come to be invalids. Divorces are not infrequent, for many will be rejected and forsaken by their husbands as I was.

Not only a victim's personal life but her ability to earn an income for herself and her family may also be sacrificed. Jobs may be lost, as well as employer-provided health insurance. The insurance policies of policy holders may be either canceled or amended to reject coverage for silicone illness. When these eventualities occur, replacement health coverage usually cannot be bought.

A majority of women are then unable to pay for their medical needs, although the cost of an explant surgery is often only the beginning of interminable medical expenses. Some might also incur medical monitoring and treatment expenses for their children. As a consequence of their implant-associated illnesses, a large percentage of silicone victims grow destitute.

Representative Joan Pitkin, who so fervently fought in the past for informed consent for implant patients, has initiated legislation to provide health insurance protection for these women. Two of Rep. Pitkin's bills, which were presented to the Maryland State House and Senate during the 1993 legislative session, have passed. One concerns the health insurance providers' disclosure of breast implant-related coverage. Another, an anti-discrimination bill, prohibits an insurer's enactment of preexisting medical consideration penalties, raises in premiums or the cancellation of insurance policies. Rep. Pitkin has currently proposed other health-related legislation to aid implant patients, and she is to be commended for her perseverance in seeking this requisite support for those so ill from silicone.

It is hoped that representatives in other states will follow suit in bringing forth their own implant-related health protection programs. Disability benefits for these injured women are also needed. Attorneys should assist implant victims in this area of financial relief. One ill implant patient in California has just received disability approval because of her physician's diagnosis of silicone poisoning.

# TORN ILLUSIONS

This is encouraging, but a long journey lies ahead before all implant patients will have the resources they so urgently need and seek.

Before this comes to pass, the only means for silicone victims to recoup their financial losses and provide for their future medical care may be filing silicone implant liability litigation. However, many people discover that this is another leap in the dark, for most are as unacquainted with the legal system as I was when I sought to file the same kind of lawsuit.

Not only does filing a lawsuit require proper information but, realistically, lawsuits involve a lot of time, often years, in order to procure financial recovery for the injured. Nevertheless, women can and often do secure compensation through the legal process. For those who have not filed an implant-related legal action, several organizations may be contacted for information, advice and assistance. One, the Association of Trial Lawyers of America (ATLA), formed a Breast Implant Litigation Group in 1989. Another, Public Citizen Health Research Group (PCHRG), sponsors a Silicone Clearinghouse for attorneys and distributes a list of their clearinghouse members. In addition, Command Trust Network supplies attorney recommendations (Appendix).

Thousands of silicone-related liability cases have already been filed, which include cases regarding gel-filled, saline and polyurethane-coated silicone implants. By January of 1993, approximately 1,300 liability cases were filed in the United States federal court alone. Within two months, this number increased by another 1,000 cases. Today, there are more than 12,000 active cases in federal courts (with an equal number pending) and upwards of 5,000 cases have been filed in state courts. Lawsuits like these continue to be initiated in the United States as well as in many other countries. For instance, Dr. Britta Ostermeyer-Shoaib of Baylor has reported that 10,000 Australian cases were filed in the United States through the Texas state courts in the fall of 1993.

In the United States implant-related legal actions may be filed in either state or federal courts according to each state's individual procedural rules. Although these rules vary among the states, the federal court rules are uniform. Diversity jurisdiction factors, which relate to the location and residence of a defendant (in this case the manufacturer), influence the choice of court filing for the plaintiff (the implant patient). If the defendant does not reside in the state of the plaintiff's filing—as routinely occurs in implant liability cases—diversity jurisdiction exists. In this event, the legal action qualifies for federal court filing.

Although lawsuits can be filed in state court despite any existing diversity factors, when a plaintiff does so the defendant acquires the right to demand that the case be removed to federal court. In essence, few dissimilarities distinguish the state and federal court proceedings. However, one difference is that federal courts require a unanimous jury verdict while some state courts do not. Because federal courts may also involve longer procedural delays due to a backlog of criminal cases, many people prefer to file their lawsuits in state courts.

The 1992 formation of the Multidistrict Litigation Panel (MDL) further encumbered many plaintiffs' progress in federal court proceedings. The panel, headquartered in Washington, reviews statistical data while watching for trends of increasing litigation pertaining to a single issue. On the exact date for which my trial was set, the Judicial Panel arrived at a determination to unify the increasing breast implant litigation. Subsequently, all federal court-filed liability cases were transferred to Judge Samuel Pointer of the Northern District of Alabama and the Judicial Panel on Multidistrict Litigation and placed under his jurisdiction. Instantly, my court date was nullified and, once again, I waited.

Despite my profound disappointment at the loss of my trial date, I felt heartened by the fact that the MDL still guaranteed the right to an individual trial by jury rather than demanding all legal actions be combined into a joint trial (a joint trial is a class action lawsuit, which involves a large number of plaintiffs who jointly pursue a legal action against a defendant). In 1992, a national class action on behalf of all implant patients had been filed in Cincinnati, Ohio. A deadline date was never issued, and the action was later incorporated into th MDL.

# TORN ILLUSIONS

The primary function of the MDL is to coordinate all pretrial aspects of implant litigation. An example is discovery, which is the process by which plaintiffs collect documents and sworn testimony from the defendants and vice-versa. The MDL's pretrial common discovery effort is under the direction of Judge Pointer, and the results of the discovery process are made available to all plaintiffs' attorneys. A central depository has been created to house these discovery documents as they are gathered. Attorneys may access the stored information through a computer data base or visit this depository to gain access to the stored documents. Thereby, the MDL consolidation greatly lessens the trial preparation expenses of individual implant litigants and their attorneys. This is the major advantage of the multidistrict coordination.

Judge Pointer further lifted all prior court-issued protective orders. The "sealing" of court documents by these orders prevented their future use. In the past, to a plaintiff's disadvantage, manufacturers had obtained court orders which had stymied the disclosure and dissemination of much decisive legal evidence. Dow Corning obtained one of the earliest protective orders after a jury returned a guilty verdict (that was soon appealed) in the 1984 Stern vs. Dow Corning court case.

During the appeal proceedings, the Stern case was settled out-of-court. However, the nondisclosure of prior court-entered evidence was a condition of settlement. Implant liability lawsuits are also often settled pre-trial. Most, if not all, of these settlements have required that plaintiffs sign a strict "gag" order (a pledge of silence), which includes the nondisclosure of information. In such settlements plaintiffs are usually awarded substantially smaller sums than they would get in a court award following a courtroom victory. For instance, Dow Corning offered Mariann Hopkins a $200,000 settlement before her 1991 trial, which she rejected. Mariann's final court award exceeded $7 million.[1]

Over the years, these protective and "gag" orders have successfully hampered the discovery process in many cases and impeded public disclosure.

Nevertheless, it is completely understandable that many women will accept pretrial settlements with these limitations in order to bring about the end to their lengthy and often agonizing litigation. In my own litigation, settlement was never an option. The defendants, Dow Corning and Heyer-Schulte, benefited from many extensions of the litigation (thus prolonging its conclusion).

From the beginning, the MDL consolidation of all federal court cases has entailed delays for victims' cases. My case was no exception. The delay kept my implant litigation in abeyance as the MDL gained momentum and fulfilled its objectives. The strived-for goal was to have court dates granted by the close of 1993. The MDL proceedings initially presented a welcomed respite for the implant industry, although any postponements derived were only temporary reprieves for the industry. Now, the collection and mutual sharing of evidence proves very effective.

Nevertheless, during the process, many in the industry continue to delay or refuse to produce and dispense corporate documents that may bring the legal battle to a close. According to one informed expert witness, many involved in the MDL coordination have suspicions that documents pertinent could have been secretly shredded and destroyed during this discovery process. At best, the implant industry is known to place roadblocks in the way of legal discovery.

Heyer-Schulte, a subsidiary of Baxter Healthcare Corporation and a defendant in my own liability litigation, informed the MDL in 1993 that the documents to be produced relating to the company's silicone studies, were too "burdensome" to locate.[2] Judge Pointer, shortly thereafter, allowed three plaintiff attorneys to enter two of the Heyer-Schulte facilities to search for the evidence. The MDL Plaintiffs' Steering Committee (PSC), a board comprised of appointed attorneys who represent the interests and concerns of plaintiffs involved in the MDL, requested that the court impose a sanction on the corporation regarding this impropriety. Judge Pointer did, in fact, respond with an order requiring Heyer-Schulte to pay the attorneys' time and costs in the amount of $55,000.[3]

# TORN ILLUSIONS

It is rumored that Dow Corning has not disclosed all the evidence in spite of Chairman Keith McKennon's pledge before the 1992 FDA advisory panel that all pertinent data required by the FDA would be released. Consequently, Dow Corning has been served with two subpoenas by the United States' Attorney's office and is currently under Federal Grand Jury investigation.[4] The Grand Jury has demanded the same documents which both the FDA and the American Trial Lawyers' Association (ATLA) seek. These include the full Griffen Bell report relevant as to whether there was falsification and replacement of oven temperature recording charts which were not revealed for many years (Chapter VI). Dow Corning hired former Attorney General, Griffen Bell, to conduct a corporate review. Before Mr. Bell completed his written report, Dow Corning had described his assignment as an "independent investigation." Later the grounds for withholding the former attorney general's commentary, then sought by many, was attorney/client privilege. Mr. Bell's job description was amended to one that encompassed "legal advice."[5]

One FDA official's statement sheds light on this situation, "Dow Corning has tried to create the public impression that they're cooperating fully with us, while they have sent us hundreds of thousands of documents that were reviewed for the [Griffen Bell] report not organized in any useful order."[6] The FDA stated that a review of the Griffen Bell report was necessary in order to correctly evaluate the data and possibly issue a public warning. To many it appears that the missing key—Mr. Bell's interpretive report—must be quite damaging to Dow Corning. Another recent incident adds to this: during state court proceedings in a 1993 Denver, Colorado trial, Dow Corning attorneys attempted to offer into evidence pieces of elastomer that were twice the thickness of their own marketed implant shell. When the difference was discovered, the presiding judge, who became discernibly annoyed, ordered the "evidence" removed from his courtroom.[7]

As defendants in implant litigation, often manufacturer's attorneys have tried to use a statute of limitations defense in order to disqualify plaintiff cases. In a number of states, statutes of limitations impose an outer time limit, which restricts one's ability to file a legal claim after the specified time period has expired. (These statutes may be overturned in some states.) However, the employment of a statute of limitations defense actually places the industry in a rather compromising position. On one hand, the defendants state that a plaintiff should have realized that the breast implants caused her injury and filed her suit earlier. On the other hand, they must deny the existence of silicone-associated illness. This seems to me a difficult position to maintain. How could women have known the implants were responsible for their injuries when even physicians had not been informed of silicone illness? I should note that in my own legal action, a federal judge did not grant Heyer-Schulte and Dow Corning a statute of limitations dismissal.

During a January 1993 silicone seminar in Florida, plaintiff attorney Dan Bolton discussed legal actions that will guard against this line of defense and protect the right to proceed with litigation in the future. (I recommend that each and every silicone-implanted woman inquire into any and all litigation positions.) Mr. Bolton described the two defensive actions; one is the filing of a dormant docket, which permits a legal action to be later implemented. Another is the filing of a medical monitoring lawsuit, which provides for an eventual rupture and/or the development of systemic illness. Individual second generation lawsuits may also be filed. A medical monitoring class action on behalf of all second generation implant victims is now in the process of being filed in New York.

Lawyers for manufacturers have subjected plaintiffs to many forms of emotional duress. The grueling six days of my own 1990 depositions, conducted by Dow Corning's Florida attorney, was the most humiliating experience of my life. I felt berated, denigrated and embarrassed. My own attorney, James McMaster of Palm Beach, stated his impression of the display presented at my deposition as the defendant's use of "intimidation and embarrassment," in an effort to force me to "flee from the room in tears" and "forego my lawsuit." However, I did not flee. Rather, I stated my objection to the abusive treatment. Although I believe that Dow Corning's legal counsel behaved extremely poorly at the deposition, the attorney representing Heyer-Schulte remained a gentleman throughout the proceedings. In response to my having gone on record voicing my displeasure over my interrogation, he was quick to disclaim any participation on his part in the use of plaintiff-directed intimidation.

According to many women with whom I have spoken, Dow Corning has the worst reputation for these tactics. This stratagem is not reserved for the plaintiff alone. My ex-husband told me that in 1992 he felt hounded and harassed by Dow Corning's attorney during a stream of telephone calls, which ended in Paul's refusal to speak further with this attorney.

Teresa, who had been my housekeeper and companion during the early years of my ordeal, also felt menaced. She told me that during the course of my litigation she was approached at her home by a detective whom she described as "rough, scary and gangster-looking." Next, the attorneys for Dow Corning and Heyer-Schulte attorneys paid Teresa—a key witness—a surprise visit. At first, Teresa said she tried to deny them entrance into her home, but the two pressed the issue and would not leave until she spoke with them. Not aware of her legal rights concerning this invasion of privacy, she nervously agreed to be interviewed.

For the most part, the alleged intimidation of plaintiffs has been ineffective. I, and thousands of others, are still standing our ground. The victims have now united to take committed action. The MDL's intention to have plaintiffs' depositions filed as a matter of record (for attorney use only) should put an end to intimidating behavior.

The preponderance of medical and legal evidence now in circulation leads me to believe that the days of courtroom confrontations as a viable option for the defense in silicone suits are rapidly dwindling. The powerful consolidation of the MDL, which can find criminal negligence, the levying of stiff punitive court awards and the assemblance of increasing silicone-related medical documentation and research, assures plaintiffs that fair legal settlement will be achieved in the near future.

In fact, this has already begun. The Breast Implant Information Foundation (BIFF) reported in their spring 1993 newsletter that Mentor Corporation has established a $24 million fund to settle their breast implant liability cases over the next four years. Mentor, the sole participant in the FDA program of restricted silicone implantation, also stated a plan to withdraw from both the FDA clinical trials and the manufacturing of silicone implants by the end of 1994. According to an April 6, 1993 article in the *Mealey's Litigation Report*, other manufacturers were in negotiation with an MDL Plaintiffs' Settlement Committee concerning their own initiation of a similar fund applicable to the "global settlement" of all breast implant litigation.[8] This information received MDL Plaintiff Committee verification at that time.[9]

After months of secretly held negotiations, Dow Corning made the unexpected announcement on September 9, 1993 of a proposal to fund a $4.75 billion "global settlement" pool.[10] The terms of this new "global settlement" proposal will most likely supersede national joint action. One news article reported that the fund is to be maintained over a thirty year period with payments from Dow Corning and other implant manufacturers, raw material suppliers, insurance companies and plastic surgeons who are being sued in connection with silicone breast implants.

Once finalized, Judge Pointer is expected to conduct fairness hearings before issuing his approval. Upon ratification, an MDL medical panel will be selected as a review board, which will classify a claimant's illness into a category in order to determine the amount of compensation. A plaintiff may elect to either opt-in or opt-out of the global settlement program; a claimant may also turn down the settlement offer and still pursue a legal action through the courts.

A review of the proposal shows the fund to be inclusive of all silicone-gel, saline and second generation implant-injured claimants. The settlement provisions extend to plaintiffs whose cases are filed in both federal and state courts, as well as to those women not actively involved in litigation. The proposal's Disease Compensation Program is divided into three main categories: Systemic Sclerosis-Scleroderma/Lupus with a $2 million cap; atypical neurological ˙syndrome/mixed connective-tissue disease/overlap syndrome/Polymyositis-Dermatomyositis with a $1.5 million cap; and atypical connective-tissue disease-atypical rheumatic syndrome/non-specific autoimmune/Sjogren Syndrome with a one million dollar cap. (Explanations are also covered.) Women who receive compensation from the fund may reenter the program at a later date when other additional implant-associated complications and illnesses develop.

Unfortunately, Dow Corning's highly publicized announcement of a $4.5 billion compensation pool to fund the settlement of implant litigation in its entirety is not the awe-inspiring settlement it appears at first. According to a statement of principle for global settlement, $1.5 billion, not $4.5, has been allocated for today's claimants.[11] The quoted $4.75 billion total will be contributed over a thirty year period without requirements for supplementary contributions. There is no doubt that the number of silicone implant cases already on record is staggering, and more will come. In a letter written to attorney Dan Bolton, a member of the Plaintiffs' Steering Committee (PSC), Dr. Norman Anderson of Johns Hopkins University School of Medicine stated a recent projection of implant-related disease costs. He reported that "very conservative estimates project total expenditures of 133 to 169 billion dollars for effective monitoring, management and rehabilitation of breast implants recipients residing in the United States alone. Thus 1.5 billion will hardly be enough to take care of today's victims."[12]

There are other shortcomings in the original proposal: reimbursement for damages arising from wage losses, pain and suffering were excluded; past disabilities are not compensated, only those which are current, younger women have higher payment schedules than older women for the same disease and cancer is not included in a scheduled category. Of great concern is the fact that the Disease Compensation Program's category, which will compensate the majority of claims concerning "atypical" illness is the least funded of the three categories proposed. Furthermore, the disease descriptions and requirements of the category in which most women will be placed, do not address the full range of silicone-associated medical conditions and illnesses as experienced by the majority of victims. Nor has it defined silicone toxicity. Rather, silicone illness, which is a specific disease of its own, has in greater part been molded to conform to the established criteria of other existing diseases. With scant reliable research having ever been conducted, silicone illness is not yet accurately labeled, nor categorized.

Regardless of what disease classification a claimant may be given, the payments listed in the schedule will then be decreased by pro-rata reductions when a category exceeds its set limit. Without question, this will happen very quickly in the "atypical" category—the one most likely to be overrun with claims. According to attorney Dan Bolton, who referred to the compensation program as "a house of cards" that may "collapse under the sheer number of claims submitted," claimants may expect payment reductions of at least twenty-five percent.[13] Many estimate that the reductions will be far higher. An appraisal of the global settlement proposal by attorney Christopher Placitella, liaison counsel for New Jersey state court silicone-breast implant litigants, is particularly alarming. Dr. Placitella states:

> If one were to assume an extremely conservative estimate of only 25,000 current claims in the atypical autoimmune disease category, $7 billion would be required to satisfy all such claims and not the $500 million currently allocated. As a result, the average claim in this category will be racheted down by more than eighty percent, and *all other claims* in the matrix will be racheted down on a pro rata basis by more than seventy percent of the value represented in the matrix.[14]

In other words, the fund will pay claimants little in actual compensation monies. Therefore, we may ask how the proposal passed with approval if reviewed by the MDL Plaintiffs' Steering Committee (PSC). The answer is, it did not. The proposal has been negotiated by a settlement committee made up of several members of the PSC and the implant industry. A letter from attorney Dan Bolton to the Plaintiff Steering Committee objected to the stealth surrounding the proposal's conception. Although a member of the PSC, Mr. Bolton was not consulted during the settlement negotiations. He has written the following:

It seems nothing short of bizarre that, after months and months of negotiations, the full PSC was first advised on Friday, September 3, of a meeting to be held in Atlanta, following the Labor Day weekend, on Tuesday morning, September 7. During the meeting, members first received limited and self-serving details about the settlement proposal.[13]

It is noted that the proposed settlement, as negotiated, did provide for the PSC's own needs with a $150 million allocation for payment of "administrative fees," which the committee will assess at its discretion. In addition, the PSC will garner six percent of each litigant's individual attorney fees and court-awarded moneys to be paid to the committee upon receipt of any settlement. This could easily amount to an astronomical payout to the PSC.

I fear that the end result of the global settlement may only be additional exploitation of already victimized women. Attorney Dan Bolton's conclusion increases my fears. His letter to the PSC stated the following:

> The legacy of the MDL 926 should not be a deceptive settlement program that ensnares women by holding out the illusion of large settlement figures. . . . I know that breast implant support groups and the victims themselves will be outraged by this sellout when they understand the fine print in this settlement proposal.[13]

The National Breast Implant Plaintiffs' Coalition—a 7,000 member organization of women involved in implant litigation—publicly denounced the presented proposal. An October 1993 letter from Gail Armstrong, the Coalition's spokesperson, notified the PSC of the organization's disapproval. She stated:

> Given the gross insufficiencies of the original proposal, and the impulsively rash manner in which it was made public, complete with inflated individual settlement figures, we must seriously question the integrity of the negotiating parties.[15]

I do not think that the proposal is fair or just. My own letter to the PSC expressed my concern and described the proposal "as enabling the ultimate betrayal of the women whose lawsuits were entrusted, beyond their control, into your care and safekeeping."

The manufacturers' proposal did not immediately receive Judge Pointer's approval; due to much opposition raised over its terms, the proposal was subjected to renegotiation.

On February 14, 1994, a new release reported that "almost all major United States makers of silicone breast implants have struck a deal over funding" for the global settlement pool. According to one negotiator, "a dozen or so critical issues" may "still pose problems, but I think it's inevitable now that there will be a deal."[16]

One month later, three of the largest implant corporations, Dow Corning, Bristol Myers-Squibb and Baxter Healthcare, as well as a number of smaller companies, announced their approval of a 3.7 billion dollar settlement fund to compensate injured implant recipients over the next thirty years.[17] Other manufacturers—including 3M and Union Carbide—are still conducting negotiations and their possible participation at a later date may eventually add an estimated one billion dollars to the settlement fund.

On April 4, United States District Judge Samuel Pointer of Birmingham, Alabama, gave his provisional approval of the newly proposed settlement agreement; final approval is expected by August.[18] In an effort to make the settlement terms more attractive to claimants, Judge Pointer restricted individual attorney fees and costs so that women would receive at least seventy-five percent of their settlement moneys. He also appointed as claims administrator State Court Judge Ann Cochran of Houston. Her appointment was applauded by national support group leader Sybil Goldrich of Command Trust, who referred to Judge Cochran as one "who understands the real issues the women have to deal with."[18]

Nonetheless, for the time being most implant patients and their attorneys remain skeptical regarding the global settlement. The past cannot be altered. The implant industry leaves behind a path of desolation and destruction. I lost over a decade of my own life to silicone illness, along with my health, husband, home and livelihood. Having shared in my losses, my children were further deprived of a mother during their formative years. They lived in constant fear that I would die.

During my 1991 deposition, Dow Corning's representative had asked me what I considered to be my greatest accomplishment. I replied that it was my success in raising two children who are stable, kind and mature adults in spite of our ordeal. The role they played in my recovery formed the foundation of the strength I needed to survive so great an affliction.

Acceptance of the hardships of these past years, of course, is made more difficult because of my acquired knowledge that silicone illness should never have occurred. Trusting by nature, my disappointments and betrayals by the people, institutions and ideals in which I placed my faith were difficult to accept. It was a painful lesson, but in the final analysis it is possible that right will triumph over wrong; if so, the implant industry will pay its debt to society.

Many women have tragically borne even worse losses than I. It is for these women and those thinking about having silicone implants that I've written this book. I would have liked to have walked away from my personal involvement in the silicone story, but I could not because of events over which I became powerless. These events took my life down roads I had not wanted to travel. Rebelling against my fate, I searched for medical answers, and slowly one ominous discovery about silicone implantation followed another until my frightening years of undiagnosed disease finally had a name—silicone illness.

After I filed my lawsuit, even more information was unearthed. Like pieces of a puzzle falling into place, the isolated bits of knowledge I gleaned over the years about the silicone tragedy came together. With my realization of the pervading horror silicone disease had caused me, once again I questioned why this had happened to me. Believing in Divine Providence, I knew there must be a reason.

I came to feel that I would not be able to go forward with my life until I wrote this book and warned others of the dangers of silicone poisoning. My book is now completed, but many tragic stories of others are only beginning. The hurt and sympathy I feel are with them; for I too have suffered.

## TORN ILLUSIONS

In the future we need to keep a vigilant watch over those in powerful positions who profit from the misery of others. We can no longer blindly trust those who greedily take so much from so many and give back nothing except false illusions, which when torn apart cause agonizing pain and deep sorrow.

I believe that those who have been victimized must seek and speak the truth, despite those who want our silence. Although as victims we all are weary, let us draw strength from one another and the joined faith which sustains us. Let us, for the sake of ourselves and others, fight on.

# AFTERWORD

*Torn Illusions* has recounted my tragic experiences with silicone. It has been a journey of survival as I fought to overcome great, if not seemingly insurmountable, odds.

From almost the beginning, the day I received silicone implants, I was besieged by a series of traumatic medical problems. To my despair, as one was solved, another appeared to take its place.

During the past fourteen years my struggle with often life-threatening medical difficulties, harrowing personal trials and drawn out legal battles have been agonizing and nearly constant.

I have lost my husband, my home, my job and much of my children's childhood to the effects of silicone poisoning.

During this time I have lived alone, without personal relationships other than those of my close family and a few loyal friends.

The silicone breast implant story is a tale of horror which has destroyed countless lives, including my own. It is a story of the seduction, betrayal and exploitation of innocent women; a story that must be told. It could have and should have been prevented.

In my opinion, the crises occurred because of corporate greed and power, subterfuge and deceit as well as a lack of interest from those who might have stopped the impending tragedy. This unwillingness to take a stand is still in evidence today.

At the same time it is also now becoming apparent that the real depth of the damage done by silicone to both men and women is just being discovered. As more and more research and medical reports surface, we are finding out that silicone devices of varied kinds, such as: penile implants, chin implants and joint replacements can cause the same life-threatening consequences that have been found to occur because of silicone breast implants. Also, we are now learning that a long period of latency—from six to twenty-six years can be associated with some long term illnesses and there is good evidence that these illnesses may be caused by silicone devices.

Thus, those like me who received silicone devices at a relatively young age may, in the future, experience the occurrence of catastrophic episodes and sicknesses or reoccurrence of, as in my case, brain seizures and/or cancer.

These are forebodings with which all of us who have had silicone implanted in our bodies must live. I have written this book because far too many silicone victims around the world do not as yet possess the information they need to gain adequate medical care and legal assistance. I hope that with enlightenment, others may be spared the physical pain and emotional agony I have suffered.

# APPENDIX

*I. Support Organizations*

*The following organizations, listed in alphabetical order, may be contacted for assistance:*

The Association of Trial Lawyers of America
Breast Implant Litigation Group
1050 31st Street NW
Washington, D.C. 20007
(800) 424-2727
Attorneys recommended for silicone implant liability litigation.

As Is, American Silicone Implant Survivors
Janet Van Winkle
1288 Cork Elm Drive
Kirkwood, MO 63122
(803) 787-5294, (314) 821-0115
Monthly newsletter: $25 yearly; send SASE.

BIIF, Breast Implant Information Foundation
Marie Walsh
P.O. Box 2907
Laguna Hills, CA 92654-2907
(714) 448-9928, FAX (714) 830-6517
Information packet: $35; Monthly newsletter: $25 yearly.

Boston Women's Health Book Collective
P.O. Box 192
West Somerville, MA 02144
(617) 625-0271, FAX (617) 625-0294
*Street address:*
240A Elm Street, 3rd Floor (Davis Square)
Somerville, MA 02144
Information packet: $10.

CATS, Children Afflicted by Toxic Substances
Jama Kim Russano
60 Oser Terrace, Suite 1
Hauppauge, NY 11788
(800) CATS-199
Second generation silicone illness; information and questionnaires.

Coalition for Silicone Survivors
Lynda Roth
P.O. Box 129
Broomfield, CO 80038-0129
(303) 469-8242, FAX: (303) 466-4084
Information packet: $5; Monthly newsletter: $25 yearly.

Command Trust Network, Nat. Breast Implant Support Group

| Augmentation: | Reconstruction: |
|---|---|
| Kathleen Anneken | Sybil Goldrich |
| P.O. Box 17082 | 256 South Linden Drive |
| Covington, KY 41017 | Beverly Hills, CA 90212 |
| (606) 331-0055 | (213 556-1738/9 |

Send $2 and SASE envelope for initial packet of information. CTN
provides a quarterly newsletter; physician and attorney
recommendations; contacts for local support groups.

# TORN ILLUSIONS

The Dayle MacIntosh Center for the Disabled
150 W. Cerritos Avenue, Building 4
Anaheim, CA 92805
(714) 772-8285
For assistance regarding social security disability refusals.

FDA, Food and Drug Administration
Consumer Affairs, HFE-88
5600 Fishers Lane
Rockville, MD 20857
(301) 443-3170, (800) 532-4440 (Hot Line)

FDA Medical Device Reporting
8757 Georgia Avenue, HF2 343
Silver Springs, MD 20910
(301) 427-7500

International Breast Implant Registry, Medic Alert, (800) 892-9211
A registry providing patient and physician notification of breast
implant-related health and safety information. First year
membership: $25; thereafter: $10 yearly.

I Know — Je Sais
Marcella Tardif                          Linda Wilson
Suite 503 Boulevard Lachapella           8316 118 Street
Montreal, Quebec H4J 2M4                 Delta, BC V4C 6H2
Canada                                   Canada
(514) 956-9735                           (604) 596-4600
An English and French support and information network.

Life After Silicone, Breast Implant Support Organization
Terry Davis                              Nina Flinn
10118 Daisy Avenue                       3901 S. Flagler St., #405
Palm Beach Gardens, FL 33410             W. Palm Bch, FL 33405
(407) 622-5469                           (407) 659-6930
Offers telephone counseling.

Maryland Women's Health Coalition
Bobbi Seabalt
1822 Notre Dame Avenue
Featherville, MD 21093
(410) 252-1545

# TORN ILLUSIONS

National Breast Implant Plaintiffs' Coalition

Gail Armstrong
3608 Drexel
Dallas, TX 75205
(214) 521-1984

Linda Hilton
2111 Lima Center Red
Chelsea, MI 48118
(313) 475-4674

National Women's Health Network
1325 G Street, NW, Lower Level
Washington, DC 20005
(202) 347-1140
Information packet: $10 (The same packer provided by
Boston Women's Health Book Collective.)

National Women's Health Resource Center
2440 M Street, NW
Washington, DC 20037
(202) 293-6045
Bi-monthly newsletter: (First copy free) $25 yearly for individuals;
$50 yearly for organizations, includes National Health Database—
Women's Health Issues.

PCHRG, Public Citizens Health Research Group
2000 P Street, NW
Washington, DC 20036
(202) 833-3000
Information packet: $6 (List of silicone clearinghouse attorney
members included.) Information packet for attorneys: $750.

Silicone Implant Awareness Support Team (SIAST)
P.O. Box 13261
Shawnee Mission, KS 66282
(913) 752-4036

Silicone Sisters Support Group
Jerrie Murphy
1621 Monterey Drive
Clearwater, FL 34616
(813) 585-4296
Information packet: $15; Newsletter: Donations welcome.

# TORN ILLUSIONS

TBIF, Texas Breast Implant Information Foundation
Coping with Breast Implants: The Support Group
P.O. Box 1426
Alief, TX 77411-1426
(713) 495-7223
Information packet: $40; telephone counseling available;
quarterly newsletter: $25 yearly.

## *II. Medical Information*

### *Silicone Breast Implant-Related Medical Testing:*

Aegis Analytical Laboratories
624 Grassmere Park, Suite 21
Nashville, TN 37211
(615) 331-5300

National Medical Services
2300 Stratford Avenue
Willow Grove, PA 19090
(215) 657-4900
Diagnostic testing to measure TDA levels in breast milk and urine.
(Have physician contact laboratory for sample collection kit.)

Antibody Assay Laboratory
1715 East Wilshire, #715
Santa Ana, CA 92705
(800) 522-2611
Silicone breast implant profile (#2876): $240
(Have physician contact laboratory for requirements.)

Balco, Bay Area Laboratory Co-Operative
1520 Gilberth Road
Burlingame, CA 94010
(415) 697-6708, (800) 777-7122
Blood serum testing for silicone analysis: $100
(Have physician contact laboratory for sample collection kit.)

Dr. Pierre Blais
Innoval Ltd.
496 Westminster Avenue
Ottawa, Ontario K2A 2V1

Canada
(613) 728-8688
FAX (613) 728-0687
Analysis of removed implants; contamination examination.

Dr. John Heggers
Shriner's Burn Institute
815 Market Street
Galvenston, TX 77550
(409) 770-6665
Silicone antibody testing.

Dr. Nir Kossovsky
UCLA
Department of Pathology
10833 Le Conte Avenue
Los Angeles, CA 90024-1732
(310) 825-0289
Silicone antibody testing; pathology tissue examination
for the presence of silicone and inflammatory responses.

Immunosciences Laboratory, Inc.
8730 Wilshire Blvd., #305
Beverly Hills, CA 90211
(310) 657-1077, (800) 950-4686, FAX (310) 657-1053
Silicone antibody testing, immunological profile and chemical
antibody testing: $550 inclusive.

Dr. Hildegarde Sacarello-Staninger
1002 Douglas Avenue
Altamonte Springs, FL 32714
(407) 862-4419
Toxicological testing for chemical poisoning.

Dr. Douglas Shanklin
University of Tennessee
899 Madison Avenue
576 Baptist Lane
Memphis, TN 38163
(901) 528-6422
Pathology tissue examination for the presence of silicone
and inflammatory responses.

# ENDNOTES

### *Chapter Two: Discovery*

1. The skin test injection was performed by Dr. Norman Orentriech on 26 October 1987 with Dow Corning silicone (medical grade).
2. Mutaz B. Habal, "The Biological Basis for the Clinical Application of Silicones," *Archives of Sugery*, 119 (1984), 843-48.
3. Transcript of the FDA General and Plastic Surgery Devices Panel Meeting held in Bethesda, Maryland on February 18-20, 1992. (Olga J. Papach, Transcription Services, 1831 Ivy Oak Square, Reston, Virginia 22090.); see also Ch. 6, notes 75-78, and 81.

### *Chapter Three: The Only One?*

1. F. Bischoff and G. Bryson, "Carcinogenesis through solid state surfaces," *Progress in Experimental Tumor Research*, 5 (1964), 85; F. Bischoff, "Carcinogenic effects of steroids," *Advances in Lipid Research*, 7 (1969), 165.
2. Testimony of Dr. Joseph A. Bellanti, President of the American College of Allergy and Immunology before the 18-20 February 1992 FDA General and Plastic Surgery Devices Panel Meeting; transcript, Ch. 2, note 3, p. 355 (Day 2) and p. 242 (Day 1).

3. T. C. Mason, "Hyperprolactinemia and galactorrhea associated with mammary prostheses and unresponsive to bromocriptine: a case report," *Journal of Reproductive Medicine*, 36 July (1991), 541-42.

4. Luis J. Jara, Carlos Lavalle, Antonio Fraga, et al., "Prolactin, immunoregulation, and autoimmune diseases," *Arthritis and Rheumatism*, 20 (5) (1991), 273-84.

5. Victor J. Selmanowitz and Norman Orentriech, "Medical-grade fluid silicone. A monographic review," *Dermatologic Surgery and Oncology*, 3 (6) (November/December) (1977), 623-36.

6. 1992 FDA General and Plastic Surgery Devices Panel Meeting transcript, Ch. 2, note 3, p. 335 (Day 2).

*Chapter Four: Awareness*

1. Human Resources and Intergovernmental Relations Subcommittee of the Committee on Government Operations, "The FDA's Regulation of Silicone Breast Implants," staff report (ISBN 0-16-039937-8), (Washington, D.C.: U. S. Printing Office, 1993), p. 3; see also Richard Ellenbogen et al., "Injectible fluid silicone therapy, human morbidity and mortality," *Journal of the American Medical Association*, 234 (1975), 308-09; Richard Ellenbogen and Leonard R. Rubin, "Toxicity associated with injectible silicone," in *Biomaterials in Reconstructive Surgery*, ed. Leonard R. Rubin (St. Louis: C. V. Mosby Company, 1983), pp. 252-259; see also notes 16 and 17.

2. J. L. Baker et al., "Positive identification of silicone in human mammary capsular tissue," *Plastic and Reconstructive Surgery*, 69 (1982), 56; Donald E. Barker, Marvin I. Retsky, and Sherill Schultz, "Bleeding of silicone from bag-gel breast implants, and its clinical relation to fibrous capsule reaction," *Plastic and Reconstructive Surgery*, 61 (1978), 836-41; Robert B. Bergman and A. E. Van der Ende, "Exudation of silicone through the envelope of gel-filled breast prostheses," *British Journal of Plastic Surgery*, 32 (1979), 31-34; G. Brandt, V. Breiting, M. Christen, et al., "Five years experience of breast augmentation using silicone gel prostheses with emphasis on capsular skrinkage," *Scandinavian Journal of Plastic Surgery*, 18 (3) (1984), 311-16; E. Domanskis and J. Owsley, "Histological investigation of the following breast augmentation," *Plastic and Reconstructive Surgery*, 58 (1976), 689; R. M. Gayou and R. Rudolph, "Capsular contracture around silicone mammary prostheses," *Annals of Plastic Surgery*, 2 (1) (1979), 62-71; Richard J. Hausner, Frederick J. Schoen, M. A. Mendez-Fenandez, et al., "Migration of silicone gel to

# TORN ILLUSIONS

auxillary lymph nodes after prosthetic mammaplasty," *Archives of Pathology and Laboratory Medicine*, 195 (1981), 371-72; Nir Kossovsky et al., "Analysis of surface morphology of recovered silicone mammary prostheses," *Plastic and Reconstructive Surgery*, 71 (6) (1983), 795-804; M. A. Mandel and D. F. Gibbon, "The presence of silicone in breast capsules," *Aesthetic Plastic Surgery*, 3 (1979), 219-225; J. Smahel, "Foreign material in the capsules around breast prostheses and the cellular reaction to it," *British Journal of Plastic Surgery*, 32 (1979), 35-42; H. Wagner et al., "Electron and light microscopy examination of capsules around breast implants," *Plastic and Reconstructive Surgery*, 60 (1979), 49; M. G. Wickham and J. L. Abraham, "Silicon identification in prosthesis-associated fibrous capsule," *Science*, 199 (1978), 437-39.

3. L. C. Argenta, "Migration of silicone gel into breast parenchyma following mammary prosthesis rupture," Aesthetic Plastic Surgery, 7 (1983), 253-54; A. Capozzi, R. DuBou, and V. R. Pennisi, "Distant migration of silicone gel from a ruptured breast implant," *Plastic and Reconstructive Surgery*, 62 (1978), 302-03; Frank McDowell, "Pop goes the breast! Capsule or implant? Beginning or end?" *Plastic and Reconstructive Surgery*, 59 (1977), 836-837; G. H. Schmidt, "Mammary implant failure," *Annals of Plastic Surgery*, 5 (5) (1980), 369-71; P. L. Schnur, "Case of the disappearing breast implants," *Plastic and Reconstructive Surgery*, 20 (1988), 270-71; L. G. Theophelis and T. R. Stevenson, "Radiographic evidence of breast implant rupture," *Plastic and Reconstructive Surgery*, 78 (1986), 673-75; see also note 5.

4. O. Asplund, "Capsular contracture in silicone gel and saline-filled breast implants after reconstruction," *Plastic and Reconstructive Surgery*, 73 (2) (1984), 270-75; Domanskis and Owsley, note 2; R. M. Gayou, "A histological comparison of contracted and noncontracted capsules around silicone breast implants," *Plastic and Reconstructive Surgery*, 63 (1979), 700-07; C. J. Hipps, D. R. Raju, and R. Straith, "Influence of some operative and post-operative factors on capsular contracture around breast implants," *Plastic and Reconstructive Surgery*, 61 (1978), 384-89; S. Hoffman, "The management of severe capsular contracture following breast augmentation," *Aesthetic Plastic Surgery*, 7 (1983), 109-12; J. O. Oaesley, "Histological investigation of etiology of capsular contracture following augmentation mammaplasty," *Plastic and Reconstructive Surgery*, 58 (1976), 689-93; F. E. M. Missotten, "Giant cyst formation in a fibrous capsule following breast augmentation. A case report and discussion on the pathology," *British Journal of Plastic Surgery*, 38 (4)

(1985), 579-82; A. B. Redfern, J. J. Ryan, and C. T. Su, "Calcification of the fibrous capsule about mammary implants," *Plastic and Reconstructive Surgery*, 59 (1977), 249-51; J. Smahel, "Foreign material in the capsules around breast prostheses and the cellular reaction to it," *British Journal of Plastic Surgery* 32 (1979), 35-42; see also Smahel, note 2; Charles A. Vinnik, "Spherical contracture of fibrous capsule around breast implants," *Plastic and Reconstructive Surgery*, 58 (1976), 555-60; C. Williams et al., "The effects of hematoma on the thickness of pseudosheaths around silicone implants," *Plastic and Reconstructive Surgery*, 56 (1975), 194.

5.  D. B. Addington and R. E. Mallin, "Closed capsulotomy causing fractures of the scar capsule and the silicone bag of a breast implant," *Plastic and Reconstructive Surgery*, 62 (1978), 300-01; H. V. Eisenberg and R. J. Bartels, "Ruptures of a silicone bag-gel breast implant by closed compression capsulotomy, case report," *Plastic and Reconstructive Surgery*, 59 (1977), 849-50; M. C. Feliberti, A. Arrillaga, and G. A. Colon, "Rupture of inflated breast implants in closed compression capsulotomy," *Plastic and Reconstructive Surgery*, 59 (6) (1977), 848; R. P. Gruber and G. Friedman, "The pressures generated by closed capsulotomies of augmented breasts," *Plastic and Reconstructive Surgery*, 62 (3) (1978), 379-80; J. M. Goin, "High-pressure injection of silicone gel into an axilla: a complication of closed compression capsulotomy of the breast," *Plastic and Reconstructive Surgery*, 62 (1978), 891; T. T. Huang, S. J. Blackwell, and S. R. Lewis, "Migration of the silicone gel after the 'squeeze technique' to rupture a contracted breast capsule," *Plastic and Reconstructive Surgery*, 61 (1978), 277-80; G. D. Nelson, "Complications of closed compression after augmentation mammaplasty," *Plastic and Reconstructive Surgery*, 66 (1980), 71-73; D. E. Tolhurst, "Nutcracker technique for compression rupture of capsules around breast implants," *Plastic and Reconstructive Surgery*, 61 (1978), 795.

6.  J. Apesos and T. L. Pope Jr., "Silicone granuloma following closed capsulotomy of mammary prosthesis," *Annals of Plastic Surgery*, 14 (5) (1985), 403-06; Argenta, note 3; E. Benjamin et al., "Silicone lymphadenopathy: a report of two cases, one with concomittant malignant lymphoma," *Diagnostic Histopathology*, 5 (2) (1982), 133-41; Caozzi, Du Bou, and Pennisi, note 3; C. Delange, J. J. Shane, and F. B. Johnson, "Mammary silicone granuloma: migration of silicone fluid to abdominal wall and inquinal region," *Archives of Dermatology*, 108 (1978), 104-07; W. C. Foster, D. S. Springfield, and K. L. B. Brown, "Pseudotumor of the arm associated with rupture of silicone-gel breast

prostheses," *The Journal of Bone and Joint Surgery*, 65A (1983), 548-551; Huang, Blackwell, and Lewis, note 5; Hausner, Schoen, and Mendez-Fernandez, note 2; Kossovsky et al., note 2; James Mason and Prapand Apisarnthanarox, "Migratory silicone granuloma," *Archives of Dermatology*, 117 (1981), 366-67; Schnur, note 3; William D. Travis, Karoly Balogh, and Jerold L. Abraham, "Silicone ganulomas: report of three cases and a review of the literature," *Human Pathology*, 16 (1985), 19-27; L. D. Troung, J. Cartwright, M. D. Goodman, and D. Wornich, "Silicone lymphadenopathy associated with augmentation mammaplasty; morphological features of nine cases," *The American Journal of Surgical Pathology*, 12 (6) (1988), 484-91; Barry F. Uretsky et al., "Augmentation mammaplasty associated with severe systemic illness," *Annals of Plastic Surgery*, 3 (1979), 445-47; W. J. Wintsch, J. Smahel, and L. Clodius, "Local and regional lymph node response to ruptured gel-filled mammary prostheses," *British Journal of Plastic Surgery*, 66 (1977), 886.

7. Selmanowitz and Orentriech, Ch. 3, note 5.
8. See note 6; see also Ch. 9, note 20.
9. See note 6.
10. N. Ben-Hur, D. L. Ballantyne, and T. D. Rees, "Local and systemic effect of dimethylpolysiloxane fluid in mice," *Plastic and Reconstructive Surgery*, 39 (1967), 423-26; N. Ben-Hur and Z. Newman, "Siliconoma - another cutaneous reaction to silicone fluid," *Plastic and Reconstructive Surgery*, 36 (1965), 629; John P. Heggers, Nir Kossovsky, R. W. Parsons, et al., "Biocompatibility of silicone implants," *Annals of Plastic Surgery*, 11 (1983), 38-45; John P. Heggers, L. Townand, I. Canady, et al., "Silicone hypersensitivity. An abnormal immunoglobulin in CSF," presented before the 34th Annual Meeting of the Plastic Surgery Research Council, Atlanta, 25 April 1991; Nir Kossovsky, John P. Heggers, and M. C. Dobson, "The bioreactivity of silicone," *CRC Critical Reviews of Biocompatibility*, 3 (1987), 53-85; Nir Kossovsky, John P. Heggers, and M. C. Dobson, "Experimental demonstration of the immunogenicity of silicone-protein complexes," *Journal of Biomedical Materials Research*, 21 (1987), 1125-33; Thomas D. Rees, D. L. Ballantyne, and G. A. Hawthorne, "Silicone fluid research. A follow-up summary," *Plastic and Reconstructive Surgery*, 46 (1970), 50-56; Thomas D. Rees, J. Platt, and D. L. Ballantyne, "An investigation of cutaneous response to dimethylpolysiloxane (silicone liquid) in animals and humans - a preliminary report," *Plastic and Reconstructive Surgery*, 35 (1965), 131-38; J. A. Lilla and L. M. Vistnes, "Long term study of reactions to various

silicone breast implants in rabbits," *Plastic and Reconstructive Surgery*, 57 (1976), 637-48; see also note 11.

11. F. D. Beggs et al., "Oleogranuloma of the breast simulating carcinoma," *Journal of the Royal Society of Medicine*, 78 (1985), 493; G. L. Brody and C. F. Frey, "Peritoneal response to silicone fluid: a histological study," *Archives of Surgery*, 96 (1968), 237-41; John E. Christ and J. B. Askew, "Silicone granuloma of the penis," *Plastic and Reconstructive Surgery*, 69 (2) (1982), 337-39; A. J. Christie, K. A. Weinberger, and M. Dietriech, "Silicone lymphadenopathy and Synovitis: complications of silicone elastomer finger joint prostheses," *Journal of the American Medical Association*, 237 (1977), 1463-64; Foster, Springfield, and Brown, note 6; Richard J. Hausner, Frederick J. S. Schoen, and K. Kendall Pierson, "Foreign-body reaction to silicone gel in axillary lymph nodes after an augmentation mammaplasty," *Plastic and Reconstructive Surgery*, 62 (1978), 381; G. A. Kozeny, A. L. Barbato, and V. K. Bansal, "Hypercalcemia associated with silicone-induced granulomas," *New England Journal of Medicine*, 311 (17) (1984), 1103-05; D. H. Kuiper, "Silicone granulomatous disease of the breast simulating cancer," *Michigan Medicine*, (March) (1973), 215-18; I. Lighterman, "Silicone granuloma of the penis. Case reports," *Plastic and Reconstructive Surgery*, 57 (1976), 517; Robert M. Nalbandian, Alfred B. Swanson, and B. Kent Maupin, "Long-term silicone implant arthroplasty: implications of animal and human autopsy findings," *Journal of the American Medical Association*, 250 (9) (1983), 1195-98; R. Rudolph et al., "Myofibroblasts and free silicon around breast implants," *Plastic and Reconstructive Surgery*, 62 (1978), 185-96; R. A. Savrin, E. W. Martin, and R. L. Ruberg, "Mass lesion of the breast after augmentation mammaplasty," *Archives of Surgery*, 114 (1979), 1423-24; J. L. Thomsen, "Histologic changes and silicone concentrations in human breast tissue surrounding silicone breast prostheses," *Plastic and Reconstructive Surgery*, 85 (1990), 38-41; Troung et al., note 6; Wickham and Abraham, note 2; Robert A. Worsing, William D. Engber, and Thomas A. Lange, "Reactive Synovitis from particulate silastic," *The Journal of Bone and Joint Surgery*, 64 (1982), 581-85; see also note 6.

12. F. Bishcoff and G. Bryson, "Carcinogenesis through solid state surfaces," *Progress in Experimental Tumor Research*, 5 (1964), 85; G. Brand, "Foreign body induced sarcomas in cancer: a comprehensive treatise," ed. F. Beeker (New York: Plenum Press, 1975) vol. I; G. Brand, "Cancer associated with asbestosis, schistosomiasis, foreign bodies, and scars," in *Cancer, A Comprehensive Treatise*, ed. F. F. Becker (New York: Plenum Publishing

Co., 1982), vol. II, 661-92; W. A. Burns, S. Kanhouwa, L. Tillman, et al., "Fibrosarcoma occurring at the site of plastic vascular graft," *Cancer*, 29 (1972), 66-72; Judith M. Digby, "Malignant Lymphoma with intranodal silicone rubber particles following metacarpophalangeal joint replacements," *Hand*, 14 (1982), 326; and *Lancet*, 2 (1981), 580; J. W. Fehrenbacher, W. Bowers, R. Strate, et al., "Angiosarcoma of the aorta associated with a dacron graft," *The Annals of Thoracic Surgery*, 32 (1981), 297-01; J. P. Hermann, S. Kanhouwa, R. J. Kelley, et al., "Fibrosarcoma of the thigh associated with a prosthetic vascular graft," *Medical Intelligence*, 284 (2) (1971), 91; A. H. M. Siddons and A. M. MacArthur, "Carcinomata developing at the site of a foreign body in the lungs," *The British Journal of Surgery*, (vol. not on copy) (1951), 542-45; J. R. Thompson and S. D. Entin, "Primary extraskeletal chondrosarcoma: report of a case arising in conjunction with extrapleural lucite ball plombage," *Cancer*, 23 (1969), 936-39; D. S. Weinburg and B. S. Maini, "Primary sarcoma of the aorta associated with vascular prosthesis: a case report," *Cancer*, 46 (1980), 398-02; P. Zafiracopoulos and A. Rouskas, "Breast cancer at site of implantation of pacemaker generator," [letter] *Lancet*, (June) (1974), 1114.

13. Harold. L. Harris, "Survery of breast implants from point of view of carcinogenesis," *Plastic and Reconstructive Surgery*, 28 (1961), 81-83.

14. Benjamin et al., note 6; Beggs et al, note 11; H. G. Bingham et al., "Breast cancer in a patient with silicone breast implants after 13 years," *Annals of Plastic Surgery*, 20 (1988), 236-37; D. G. Bowers and C. B. Radlauer, "Breast cancer after prophylactic subcutaneous masectomies and reconstruction with silastic prostheses," *Plastic and Reconstructive Surgery*, 44 (1969), 541-44; P. E. Burns, "Breast prosthesis," [letter to the editor] *Lancet*, (December 20) (1975), 1259-60; Judith M. Digby and A. L. Wells, "Malignant lymphoma with intranodal refractile particles after insertion of silicone prostheses," [letter] *Lancet*, 2 (July-September) (1981), 580; V. Gottlieb, A. G. Muench, D. Rich, et al., "Carcinoma in augmented breasts: case reports," *Annals of Plastic Surgery*, 12 (1984), 67-69; Hausner, Schoen, Mendez-Fernandez, et al., note 2; Hausner, Shoen, and Pierson, note 11; W. C. Hueper, "Cancer induction by polyurethane and polysilicone plastics," *Journal of the National Cancer Institute*, 33 (1964), 1005-27; J. E. Hoopes, M. T. Edgerton, and W. Shelley, "Organic synthetics for augmentation mammaplasty: their relationship to cancer," *Plastic and Reconstructive Surgery*, 39 (1967), 26369; M. Johnson and H. Lloyd, "Bilateral breast cancer 10 years after augmentation

mammaplasty," *Plastic and Reconstructive Surgery*, 53 (1974), 88-90; J. Marchant, "Breast prostheses", [letter to the editor] *Lancet*, 360 (16 February) (1976); M. A. Mendez-Fernandez et al., "Paget's disease of the breast after subcutaneous masectomies and reconstruction with silastic prostheses," *Plastic and Reconstructive Surgery*, 65 (1980), 683-85; L. Morgenstern, S. H. Gleischman, S. L. Michel, et al., "Relationship of free silicone to human breast carcinoma," *Archives of Surgery*, 120 (5) (1985), 573-77; Travis, Balogh, and Abraham, note 6.

15. Morgenstern, Gleischman, Michel, et al., note 14.

16. B. R. Celli and D. M. Kovnat, "Acute pneumonitis after subcutaneous injections of silicone," [letter to the editor] *New England Journal of Medicine*, (October 6) (1983), 856-57; J. Chastre, F. Basset, and F. Viau, "Acute pneumonitis after subcutaneous injection of silicone in transsexual men," *New England Journal of Medicine*, 308 (1983), 764; Ellenbogen et al., Ellenbogen and Rubin, note 1; Y. Kobayashi, "A case of stromal sarcoma of the breast occurring after augmentation mammaplasty," *Gan No Rinsho, Japanese Journal of Cancer Clinics*, 34 (1988), 467-72; C. M. Lewis, "Inflammatory carcinoma of the breast following silicone injections," *Plastic and Reconstructive Surgery*, 66 (1980), 134-46; Mary H. McGrath and Boyd R. Burkhardt, "The safety and efficacy of breast implants for augmentation mammaplasty," *Plastic and Reconstructive Surgery*, 74 (1984), 550-60; J. M. Manresa and F. Manresa, "Silicone pneumonitis," *Lancet*, 2 (1983), 1373-75; B. Milojevic, "Complications after silicone injection therapy in aesthetic plastic surgery," *Aesthetic Plastic Surgery*, 6 (1982), 203-06; T. Naruke, "Breast cancer in patients after injection of synthetic materials into the breast for cosmetic purposes," *Japanese Medical Report*, (1970) and *Bulletin*, (1972); F. Ortiz-Monasterrio and I. Trigoss, "Management of patients with complications from injections of foreign materials into chest," *Plastic and Reconstructive Surgery*, 50 (1972), 42-47; V. R. Pennisi, "Obscure carcinoma encountered in subcutaneous masectomy in silicone and parafin-injected breasts: two patients," *Plastic and Reconstructive Surgery*, 74 (1984), 535-38; R. Raszewski et al., "A severe fibrotic reaction after cosmetic liquid silicone injection. A case report," *Journal of Cranio-Maxillo-Facial Surgery*, 18 (1990), 225-28; S. C. Symmers, "Silicone mastitis in 'topless' waitresses and some other varieties of foreign body mastitis," *British Medical Journal*, 3 (1968), 19-25; G. A. Timberlake and G. R. Looney, "Adenocarcinoma of the breast associated with silicone injections," *Journal of Surgical Oncology*, 32 (1986), 79-81; Travis, Balogh, and Abraham, note 6; Charles

A. Vinnik, "The hazards of silicone injections," [letter] *Journal of the American Medical Association*, 263 (1976), 959; T. F. Wilkie, "Late development of granuloma after liquid silicone injections," *Plastic and Reconstructive Surgery*, 60 (1977), 179; see also note 21.

17. Ellenbogen and Rubin, note 1; see also H. H. McCardy and E. T. Solomons, "Forensic examination of toxicological specimens for dimethylpolysiloxane (silicone oil)," *Journal of Analytical Toxicology*, 1 (1977), 221; cited in Marc Lappe, *Chemical Deceptions* (San Francisco: Sierra Club Books, 1991), p. 161.

18. "The FDA's regulation of silicone breast implants," note 1; see also Sidney M. Wolfe, *Women's Health Alert* (Reading, Massachusetts: Addison-Wesley Publishing Company, Inc., 1991), p. 32.

19. Reported at the 1992 Association of Trial Lawyers of America (ATLA) Breast Implant Group Seminar held at the Boca Raton Hotel and Country Club, Boca Raton, Florida. Summary memorandum dated 23 January 1992, item 43.

20. Documents presented before the FDA General and Plastic Surgery Devices Panel Meeting held on 18-20 February 1992, Bethesda, Maryland. (Transcript provided by Olga J. Papach Transcription Services, 1831 Ivy Oak Square, Reston, VA 22090), pp. 426-28 (Day 2) and p. 386 (Day 1).

21. K. Miyoshi, T. Miyamura, Y. Kobayshi, et al., "Hypergammaglobulnemia by prolonged adjuvanticity in man. Disorders developed after augmentation mammaplasty," *Japanese Medical Journal*, 2122 (1964), 9-14; see also Yasuo Kumagai, Chiyuki Abe, T. Hirano, et al., "Mixed connective tissue disease after breast augmentation which terminated in scleroderma kidney," *Rhyumachi* 21 (1981), 171-76; Yasuo Kumagai, Chiyuki Abe, and Yuichi Shiokawa, "Scleroderma after cosmetic surgery - 4 cases of human adjuvant disease," *Arthritis and Rheumatism*, 22 (1979), 532-37; Yasuo Kumagai, Yuichi Shiokawa, T. A. Medsger, et al., "Clinical spectrum of connective tissue disease after cosmetic surgery," *Arthritis and Rheumatism*, 27 (1984), 1-12; Y. Miyoshi, H. Shiragami, and K. Yoshida, "Adjuvant disease of man," *Clinical Immunology* (Tokyo), 5 (1973), 785-94; Y. Okano, M. Nishikai, and A. Sato, "Scleroderma, primary biliary cirrhosis, Sjogren's syndrome after cosmetic breast augmentation with silicone injection: a case of possible human adjuvant disease," *Annals of Rheumatic Diseases*, 43 (1984), 520-25; K. Yoshida, "Post mammaplasty disorder as an adjuvant disease of man," *Japanese Medical Journal*, 29 (1973), 318.

22. Randall M. Goldblum, Ronald P. Pelley, Alice A. O'Donell, Debra C. Pryon, and John P. Heggers, "Antibodies to silicone elastomers and reactions to ventriculoperitoneal shunts," *Lancet,* 340 (1992), 510-13; Ronald P. Pelley, John P. Heggers, and Ronald M. Goldblum, "Immunogloulins binding to polydimethylsiloxane 'silastic' tubing in the serum of children with ventriculsperitoreal shunt," Conference on the Silicone in Medical Devices, Baltimore, Maryland, 1 February 1991; see also R. B. Snow and Nir Kossovsky, "Hypersensitivity reaction associated with sterile ventriculoperitoneal shunt malfunction," *Surgical Neurology,* 31 (3) (1989), 209-14; Ron Winslow, "Silicone found to spur output of antibodies, researchers say," *Wall Street Journal,* 28 August 1992, sec. B, p. 2.

23. A. C. Allison, J. S. Harington, and M. Birbeck, "An examination of the cytotoxic effect of silica on macrophages," *Journal of Experimental Medicine,* 124 (1966), 141-53; R. W. I. Kessel, L. Monaco, and M. A. Marichisio, "The specificity of the cytotoxic action of silica: a study in vitro," *British Journal of Experimental Pathology,* 44 (1962), 351-64.

24. In press; see also Ch. 6, notes 58-62, and Ch. 7, notes 15 and 16.

25. Food and Drug Administration, *Federal Register,* 55 no. 96, 17 May 1990, p. 20571, states: "Silicone gel-filled breast implants also contain silica as a filler in the device envelopes and gels." Listed references: T. J. Haley, "Biocompatibility of monomers," in *Systemic Aspects of Biocompatibility,* ed. D. F. Williams (Boca Raton, FL: CRC Series in Biocompatibility), II, 59-90; Redinger Van Aken et al., "Silicone gel filled prosthesis," U. S. patent no. 4,455,691, June 26, 1984; see also R. S. Ward et al., "Procurement of primary referral materials," National Technical Information Service Report no. N01-HV-9-2933-5 (Washington, D.C.: GPO, 1984), cited in Marc Lappe, *Chemical Deceptions* (San Francisco: Sierra Club Books, 1991), p. 155.

26. S. A. Van Nunen, P. A. Gatenby, and A. Basten, "Post-mammaplasty connective tissue disease," *Arthritis and Rheumastism,* 25 (1982), 694-97; see also C. M. Baldwin Jr. and E. N. Kaplan, "Silicone-induced human adjuvant disease?" *Annals of Plastic Surgery,* 10 (1983), 270-73; S. J. Brozena, N. A. Fenke, C. W. Cruse, et al., "Human adjuvant disease following mammaplasty," *Archives of Dermatology,* 124 (September) (1988), 1383-86; R. A. Bryon, V. A. Venning, and A. G. Mowat, "Post-mammaplasty human adjuvant disease," *British Journal of Rheumatology,* 23 (3) (1984), 227-29; L. P. Endo, N. L. Edwards, S. Longley, et al., "Silicone and rheumatic diseases," *Seminars in Arthritis*

*and Rheumatism*, 17 (1987), 112-18; K. M. Fock, P. H. Feng, and B. H. Tey, "Autoimmune disease developing after augmentation mammaplasty: report of 3 cases," *Journal of Rheumatology*, 11 (1984), 98-100; Yasuo Kumagi, Yuichi Shiokawa, T. A. Medsger, et al. "Clinical spectrum of connective tissue disease after cosmetic surgery," *Arthritis and Rheumatism*, 27 (1) (1984), 1-12; F. J. Guitierrez and L. R. Espinoza, "Progressive systemic sclerosis complicated by severe hypertension: a reversal after silicone implant removal," *American Journal of Medicine*, 89 (3) (September) (1990), 390-92; P. E. Marik, A. L. Karl, and A. Zambakider, "Scleroderma after silicone augmentation mammaplasty. A report of two cases," *South African Medical Journal*, 77 (4) (February) (1990), 212-13; Harry Spiera, "Scleroderma after silicone augmentation mammaplasty," *Journal of the American Medical Association*, 260 (2) (1988), 236-38; Thomas J. Sergott, Joseph P. Limoli, Curtis M. Baldwin, and Donald R. Laub, "Human adjuvant disease, possible autoimmune disease after silicone implantation: a review of the literature, case studies, and speculation for the future," *Plastic and Reconstructive Surgery*, 78 (1986), 104-114; Barry F. Uretsky, James J. O'Brien, and Eugene H. Courtiss, "Augmentation mammaplasty associated with severe systemic illness," *Annals of Plastic Surgery*, 3 (1979), 445-47; Frank W. Walsh, David A. Solomon, Luis R. Espinosa, et al., "Human adjuvant disease - a new cause of chylous effusions," *Archives of Internal Medicine*, 149 (1989), 1194-96; Steven R. Weiner, P. J. Clements, and Harold E. Paulus, "Connective tissue disease after augmentation mammaplasty," *Arthritis and Rheumatism*, 32 (1989), 23-24; Steven R. Weiner and Harold E. Paulus, "Chronic arthropathy occurring after augmentation mammaplasty," *Plastic and Reconstructive Surgery*, 77 (1986), 185-87; M. H. Weisman, T. R. Vecchione, D. Albert, et al., "Connective-tissue disease following breast augmentation: a preliminary test of the human adjuvant disease hypothesis," *Plastic and Reconstructive Surgery*, 82 (1988), 626-30.

27. John Varga, H. Ralph Schumacher, and Sergio A. Jimenez, "Systemic sclerosis after augmentation mammaplasty with silicone implants," *Annals of Internal Medicine*, 111 (5) (September) (1989), 377-83.

28. Uretsky et al., note 6.

29. P. Berrino et al., "Long lasting complications with the use of polyurethane-covered breast implants," *British Journal of Plastic Surgery*, 39 (4) (1986), 549-53; William M. Cocke et al., "Foreign body reactions to polyurethane covers of some breast prostheses," *Plastic and Reconstructive*

*Surgery,* 56 (1975), 527-30; Michael E. Jabaley and Suman K. Das, "Late breast pain following reconstruction with polyurethane-covered implants," *Plastic and Reconstructive Surgery,* 78 (1986), 390-95; J. L. A. Robertson, "Late deterioration of silicone foam breast implants (case report)," *Plastic and Reconstructive Surgery* 62 (1978), 193; Leonard R. Rubin, "Degradation of the saline-filled silicone-bag breast implant," in *Biomaterials in Reconstructive Surgery,* ed. Leonard R. Rubin (St. Louis: C.V. Mosby Company, 1983), pp. 260-72; J. Smahel, "Tissue reactions to breast implants coated with polyurethane," *Plastic and Reconstructive Surgery,* 61 (1982), 80-85; Atel Vargas, "Shedding of silicone particles from inflated breast implants," [letter] *Plastic and Reconstructive Surgery,* 64 (1979), 252-53.

30. Figure quoted in an FDA memorandum written by Ronald J. Lorentzen, PhD, Executive Secretary, Cancer Assessment Committee, FDA dated 29 September 1988; information provided by Public Citizen Health Research Group (PCHRG); see also Warren E. Leary, "Breast implants, a look at the record," *New York Times,* 13 November 1988, cited in Marc Lappe, *Chemical Deceptions,* note 26, p. 158.

## *Chapter Five: Investigation*

1. Public Health Services, "Safety of silicone breast prostheses," *FDA Drug Bulletin,* February 1989; adverse reaction report (Drugs and Biologic) form FDA 1639 (7-86), U. S. Food and Drug Administration, Rockville, Maryland 20857.

2. Summaries of FDA transcripts of General and Plastic Surgery Devices Panel Meetings provided by Public Citizen Health Research Group (PCHRG) through the Silicone Clearinghouse.

3. Dr. Jenny discussed the 1978 FDA panel reviews during his presentation before the State of Florida Silicone Seminar, Tampa, Florida, 23 January 1993.

4. Food and Drug Administration, *Federal Register,* vol. 55 no. 96 FR 20569, 17 May 1990. Reference cited: *Federal Register,* 47 FR 2820-21, 19 January 1982.

5. Food and Drug Administration, *Federal Register,* 53 FR 23874, 24 June 1988, final rule reclassifying silicone gel-filled breast implants into Class III, 21 CFR 8786.3540.

6. An FDA discussion paper dated 3 November 1988; reference cited by Dr. Sidney M. Wolfe of PCHRG (#1149) during testimony given before the 22 November 1988 FDA Advisory Committee on General and Plastic

# TORN ILLUSIONS

Surgery Devices. See also *FDA Drug Bulletin*, note 1. Reference: McGrath and Burkhardt, Ch. 4, note 16.

7. Summaries of the 22 November 1988 FDA General and Plastic Surgery Devices Panel Meeting provided by PCHRG.

8. Summaries, note 7.

9. Food and Drug Administration, *Federal Register*, 56 (69), 10 April 1991, pp. 14620-14627, issued a final rule that silicone breast implant manufacturers must submit pre-market approval applications within 90 days.

10. Associated Press, "Company's breast implant data faulted," *Los Angeles Times*, 14 November 1991.

11. Lorentzen, FDA memorandum, Ch. 4, note 30.

12. PCHRG *News Release* dated 2 January 1992.

13. Excerpts and quotes from the 13-14 November 1991 FDA panel review are discussed in a 30 December 1991 letter to Commissioner David A. Kessler from Dr. Sidney M. Wolfe and Jerry Kuester of PCHRG; re: Silicone gel-filled mammary prostheses - pre-market approval.

14. "The FDA's regulation of silicone breast implants," a December, 1992, staff report (15BN 0-16-039937-8) following a three year investigation of the FDA by the Human Resources and Intergovernmental Relations Subcommittee of the Committee on Government Operations (Washington, D.C.: U. S. Printing Office, 1993), pp. 13 and 49.

15. David Hancock, "Surgeons told to halt silicone shots," *Miami Herald*, 5 February 1992, sec. B, p. 2; F. McDowell, "Complications with silicone - what grade of silicone? How do we know it was silicone?" [Editorial] *Plastic and Reconstructive Surgery*, 61 June (1978), 892-95.

16. *Federal Register*, note 4.

17. A memorandum entitled, " Review of toxicity data for silicone gel," from Robert L. Sheridan, Office of Device Evaluation, FDA to Arthur R. Norris, National Center for Toxicological Research, FDA dated 28 July 1988, cited in Sidney M. Wolfe, *Women's Health Alert* (Reading, Massachusetts: Addison-Wesley Publishing Company, Inc., 1991), p. 34.

18. A memorandum entitled, "Analysis of Dow Corning data regarding carcinogenicity of silicone gels," from Dr. D. E. Stratmeyer, Activity Chief, Health Science Branch, Center for Devices and Radiological Health, FDA, to Director, Office of Science and Technology, Center Devices and Radiological Health, dated 9 August 1988, cited in Sidney M. Wolfe *Women's Health Alert*, p. 23.

19. Food and Drug Administration, *Federal Regiser,* (21 CFR part 878) 55 (96), 17 May 1990, p. 20571. References: Benjamin et al., Ch. 4, note 6; Bingham et al., Bowers and Radlauer, Digby and Wells, Johnson and Lloyd, Marchant, and Travis, Ch 4, note 14.

20. Dr. Luu's recommendations were discussed in a 9 November 1988 letter to FDA Commission Frank Young from Dr. Sidney M. Wolfe of PCHRG (#1143). Memorandum entitled, "Master file silicone Dow Corning," from Dr. Hoan My Do Luu of the FDA Task Force dated 13 August 1988.

21. *Federal Register,* note 20, p. 20570.

22. Dr. Sidney M. Wolfe used the DES experience as an example of the importance of animal study results during testimony before the 22 November 1988 FDA Advisory Panel Meeting; see also Ch. 8.

23. M. Bibbo et al., "Follow-up study of male and female offspring of DES-exposed mothers," *Obstetrics and Gynecology,* 49 (1977), 1-8, cited in Marc Lappe, *Chemical Deceptions* (San Fransisco: Sierra Club Books, 1991), p. 155.

24. Brian Haugh, "Hollywood Panics," *The Star,* 18 December 1990, pp. 20-21.

25. "Breast implant award," *National Law Journal,* 25 March 1991; E. Frost, "Breast implant cancer link alleged," *ABA Journal,* June 1991, p. 18.

26. J. Autian et al., "Carcinogenesis from polyurethanes," *Cancer Review,* 35 (1975), 1591-96; W. C. Hueper, "Experimental production of cancer by means of polyurethane plastic," *American Journal of Clinical Pathology,* 34 (1960), 328-33; W. C. Heuper, "Cancer induction by polyurethane and polysilicone plastics," *Journal of the National Cancer Institute,* 33 (1964), 1005-27; The International Agency for Research on Cancer, "2, 4 - and 2, 6 Toulene Diisocynates," *IARC Cancer Review, IARC Monographs on the Evaluation of the Carcinogenic Risk of Chemicals to Man,* 16 (1978), 83, and 19 (1979), 303; NCI/NTP Carcinogenesis Technical Report, "Bioassay of 2, 4 Diaminotoluene for possible carcinogencitiy," (CAS no. 95-80-7, NCI-CG-TR-162), U. S. Department of Health and Human Services, 162 (1979).

27. Nancy Benac, "FDA accused of down-playing possible breast implant risk," *Orange County Register,* 28 April 1991, sec. A, p.6.

28. Benjamin E. Thysen et al., "Reproductive toxicity of 2, 4-Toluenediamine in the rat: spermatogenic and hormonal effects," *Journal of Toxicology and Environmental Health,* 16 (1985), 763-69; D. R. Varman, "Epidemiological and experimental studies on the effect of methyl

isocyanate on the course of pregnancy," *Environmental Health Prospectives*, 72 (1987), 153-57; Santosh K. Varma et al., "Reproductive toxicity of 2, 4-Toluenediamine in the rat. 3 effects on androgen-binding protein levels, selected semiferous tubule characteristics and spermatogenesis, "*Journal of Toxicology and Environmental Health*, 25 (4) (1988), 435-51.

29. "The FDA's regulation of silicone breast implants," note 14.
30. The FDA's regulation of silicone breast implants. Reference: G. Kessler, J. D. Cooper, and W. Fee, the implant industry *Newsday*, 19 January 1992.
31. Letter to Rep. John D. Dingell, Chairman, House Oversight and Investigations Subcommittee, Washington, D.C., dated 3 August 1989; PCHRG publication #1177.
32. Gina Kolata, "Consumer groups, officials question FDA's power to protect the public," *New York Times*, 26 January 1992; (*New York Times*), "Consumer groups, officials question FDA's power to protect the public," Ft. Lauderdale *Sun Sentinel*, 26 January 1992; Testimony of Dr. Sidney M. Wolfe, Director of PCHRG, before the 18-20 February 1992 FDA General and Plastic Surgery Devices Advisory Committee: Hearing on Silicone Gel Implants, PCHRG release (#1255); transcript, Ch. 2, note 3, pp. 433-34 (Day 2).
33. Tim M. Smart, "Breast Implants: What did the industry know and when?" *Business Week*, 10 June 1991, pp. 94-98.
34. Michael Castleman, "Woman's Warrior," *California Lawyer*, March 1991, pp. 45-48.
35. Nicholas Regush, "Toxic Breasts," *Mother Jones*, January/February 1992, pp.25-31; M. Kircher, *Medical Economics*, 66 (1989), 109; see also Smart, note 33.
36. "The FDA's regulation of silicone breast implants," note 14.
37. Philip J. Hilts, "Top manufacturers of breast implant replaces its chief," *New York Times*, 11 February 1992, sec. A, p. 1.
38. Leary, Ch. 4, note 30.

## *Chapter Six: Evidence Becomes Available*

1. Transcript of the FDA General and Plastic Surgery Devices Panel Meeting held in Bethesda, Maryland on February 18-20, 1992. (Olga J. Papach, Transcription Services, 1831 Ivy Oak Square, Reston, Virginia 22090.)
2. transcript, p. 21 (Day 1).
3. transcript, p. 432 (Day 2).

4. transcript, p. 109 (Day 1).
5. transcript, p. 25 (Day 1).
6. transcript, p. 75 (Day 1).
7. transcript, pp. 41-42 (Day 1).
8. transcript, p. 43 (Day 1); see also *New York Times* byline, "Implants said to rupture more often," Ft. Lauderdale *Sun-Sentinel*, 19 February 1992, sec. A, p. 3.
9. 1992 Federal Panel Review transcript, note 1, p. 45 (Day 1).
10. transcript, p. 45 (Day 1).
11. transcript, p. 46 (Day 1).
12. transcript, p. 46 (Day 1).
13. Christopher Scanlan, "Documents detail implants' hazards," *Miami Herald*, 11 February 1992, sec. A, p. 1.
14. 1992 FDA Panel Review transcript, note 1, p. 48 (Day 1).
15. transcript, p. 48 (Day 2).16. transcript, p. 50 (Day 1); Dow Corning letter to R. Kelley from D. Petraitis concerning "Bleed studies for Dr. [name omitted]," dated 26 March 1977.
16. 1992 FDA Panel Review Transcript, p. 50 (Day 1), Dow Corning letter to R. Kelley from D. Petraitis concerning "Bleed studies for Dr. [name omitted]," dated 26 March 1977.
17. See Ch. 4, note 26.
18. 1992 FDA Panel Review transcript, note 1, p. 519 (Day 2).
19. transcript, pp. 516-17 (Day 2).
20. transcript, p. 386 (Day 1); The Dow Corning study is entitled "Immunologic Enhancing Activities of Organosilicone Compounds and Non-Functioning Fluids."
21. Laura Grimmer, "Report: Dow implant files were altered," *Memphis Commerical Appeal*, 3 November 1992; Tim M. Burton, "Dow Corning employees falsified data on breast implants, counsel concludes," *Wall Street Journal*, 3 November 1992.
22. Philip J. Hilts, "Maker of implants balked at testing, its record shows," *New York Times*, 13 January 1992, p. 1; see also 1992 FDA Panel transcript, note 1, p. 51 (Day 1).
23. Reported in Attorney Dan Bolton's letter to Commissioner Kessler, dated 30 December 1991; re: Mariann Hopkins vs. Dow Corning Corporation.
24. 1992 FDA Panel Review transcript, note 1, p. 52 (Day 1).
25. *Sun Sentinel* wire service, "Breast implant maker replaces its chief," The Fort Lauderdale *Sun Sentinel*, 11 February 1992.

26. Ester Rome, "Are breast implants safe?" *Sojourner: The Women's Forum,* November 1989; published in *CTN Newsletter* (Command Trust Network), ed. Kathleen Anneken, Covington, Kentucky, Winter 1989.

27. Tim M. Burton, "Several firms face breast-implant woes," *Wall Street Journal,* 23 January 1992, sec. B, p. 1.

28. Burton.

29. Burton.

30. Bolton, note 23.

31. 1992 FDA Panel Review transcript, note 1, p. 515 (Day 2).

32. transcript, p. 201 (Day 2).

33. Studies entitled: "Histopathological examinations of wistar rats" (Table 1-3, 21 September 1968, pp. 000903-000906); "Histopathological examination of sherman rats" (Table 4, 21 September 1968, p. 00097); "Histopathological examinations of rats" (Table 5, 17 June 1968, p. 000908); "Histopathological examination of wistar rats" (Table 6, 12 October 1968, p. 000909). "Histopathological examination of fisher rats" (Table 7, 6 October 1968, p. 000910); "Histopathological examinations of wistar rats" (Table 8, 23 March 1968, p. 000911); "Histopathological examination of mice" (Table 9, 25 February 1968, p. 000912); "Histopathological examinations of mice" (Table 10, 21 October 1967, p. 000913); "Histopathological examinations of mice" (Table 11, 25 February 1968, p. 000914).

34. Histopathological studies, Table 11, 25 February 1968, p. 000914 (FDRL ref. 26F).

35. 1992 FDA Panel Review transcript, note 1, pp. 144-45 (Day 2).

36. transcript, p. 430 (Day 2); see also Chapter 5 and Chapter 8 for further information.

37. 1992 FDA Panel Review transcript, note 1, p. 88 (Day 1).

38. Dow Corning Report #47391, p. 24. Reference: A. J. Lentz, M. L. Chandler, and R. R. Levier, report 151: "Biological evaluation of an implanted silicone gel: summary of acute and chronic studies," Dow Corning TIS Report 4856, series 10030, project no. 9581, dated 17 May 1978; see also 1992 FDA Panel Review transcript, note 1, pp. 84-91 (Day 1).

39. Dow Corning Report #473915, p. 25. Reference: W. F. Boley and M. A. Bejarano, report 150: "Fate of Q7-2159A gel injected subdermal in rats: macro observations," series 1-0740, project no. 7010, data omitted.

40. FDA Panel Review transcript, note 1, p. 380 (Day 1).

41. transcript, p. 379 (Day 1).

42. transcript, pp. 164-65 (Day 2).

43. Associated Press, "Dow Corning tests reportedly hinted silicone could effect the immune system," *Orange County Register*, 20 January 1992.

44. Philip J. Hilts, "Strange history of silicone held many warning signs," *New York Times*, 18 January 1992.

45. 1992 FDA Panel Review transcript, note 1, p. 375 (Day 1).

46. transcript, p. 144 (Day 2).

47. transcript, p. 513 (Day 2).

48. transcript, pp. 384-85 (Day 1).

49. transcript, pp. 114-15 (Day 1).

50. transcript, p. 99 (Day 1).

51. transcript, p. 73 (Day 2); p. 163 (Day 2); p. 221 (Day 2); pp. 368-69 (Day 1).

52. transcript, p. 163 (Day 2).

53. transcript, p. 277 (Day 2).

54. transcript, pp. 89-91 (Day 1).

55. transcript, pp. 242-43 (Day ).

56. transcript, p. 356 (Day 2).

57. P. Ellman and R. E. Ball, "Rheumatoid disease with joint and pulmonary manifestation," *British Medical Journal*, 2 (1943), 816-20; K. Honda et al., "HLA and Silicosis in Japan," New *England Journal of Medicine*, 319 (1988); G. P. Rodnan et al., "The association of progressive systemic sclerosis (scleroderma) with coal miners' pneumoconiosis and other forms of silicosis," *Annals of Internal Medicine*, 66 (1966), 323-28; S. Suzuki, "Chest disorders and rheumatoid arthritis," *Ryumachi*, 10 (1970), 20-26; cited in Marc Lappe, *Chemical Deceptions*, Ch. 4, note 17, p. 163; see also: T. Gough, D. Rivers, and R. M. E. Seals, "Pathological studies of modified pneumoconiosis in coal miners with rheumatoid arthritis (Caplan's Syndrome)," *Thorax*, 10 (1955), 9-18; Yasuo Kumagai, Chiyuki Abe, and Yuichi Skiokawa, "Scleroderma after cosmetic surgery: four cases of human adjuvant disease," *Arthritis and Rheumatism*, 22 (1979), 532-37; Yasuo Kumagai, Yuichi Shiokawa, T. A. Medsger, and G. P. Rodnam, "Clinical spectrum of connective tissue disease after cosmetic surgery," *Arthritis and Rheumatism*, 27 (1984), 1-12; A. G. Rickards and G. M. Barnett, "Rheumatoid lung changes associated with asbestos," *Thorax*, 13 (1958), 185-92; Harry Spiera, "Scleroderma after silicone augmentation mammaplasty," *The Journal of the American Medical Association*, 260 (1988), 236-38.

58. R. M. Silver, E. E. Sahn, J. O. Allen, et al., "Demonstration of silicon in site of connective-tissue disease in patients with silicone-gel breast implants," *Archives of Dermatology*, 129 (1993), 63-68; see also E. E. Sahn, P. D. Garen, R. M. Silver, and J. C. Maize, "Scleroderma following augmentation. A report of a case and a review of the literature," *Archives of Dermatology*, 126 (9) (1990), 1198-202.

59. *Federal Register*, Ch. 4, note 26.

60. Ward et al., Ch 4, note 26.

61. 1992 FDA Panel Review transcript, note 1, p. 278 (Day 1).

62. transcript, p. 355 (Day 2); see also p. 242 (Day 1).

63. transcript, p. 74 (Day 2); see also C. H. Kirpatrick, "Delayed hypersensitivity," in *Immunological Diseases*, ed. Max Samter (Boston: Little, Brown and Company, 1988), pp. 261-277; F. J. Dixon, C. G. Cochrane and A. N. Theofilopoulus, "Immune Complex Injury," in *Immunological Diseases*, pp. 233-260.

64. Dr. Ira Finegold reported the findings of his research study in a paper presented to the November 1993 annual meeting of the American College of Allergy and Immunology, Atlanta, Georgia; Ira Finegold, "The clinical spectrum of silicone associated disease (S.A.D.)," publication pending, June 1994.

65. transcript, p. 31 (Day 1).

66. transcript, p. 240 (Day 1).

67. transcript, p. 253 (Day 1).

68. transcript, p. 331 (Day 1); see also Frank B. Vasey, D. L. Havice, T. S. Bocanegra, et al., "Clinical manifestations of fifty consecutive women with silicone breast implants and connective tissue disease," *Arthritis and Rheumatism*, 35 (1992), S21; Frank B. Vasey, T. S. Bocanegra, D. L. Havice, et al., "Silicone associated with connective tissue disease: onset of systemic signs and symptoms after traumatic rupture of silicone gel filled breast implants," *Arthritis and Rheumatism*, 35 (1992), S24.

69. transcript, p. 261 (Day 1); see also Steven R. Weiner and Harold E. Paulus, "Chronic arthropathy occurring after augmentation mammaplasty," *Plastic and Reconstructive Surgery*, 77 (1986), 185-87.

70. Kumagai, Shiokawa, Medsger, and Rodnam, note 57.

71. Spiera, note 57.

72. 1992 FDA Panel Review transcript, note 1, p. 269 (Day 1).

73. transcript, pp. 275-276 (Day 1).

74. transcript, p. 276 (Day 1).

75. transcript, pp. 281-282 (Day 1).

76. transcript, p. 285 (Day 1).
77. transcript, p. 287 (Day 1).
78. Reported by Linda Hilton of "Right to Know," Ann Arbor, Michigan, published in *B.I.F.F. Newsletter* (Breast Implant Information Foundation), ed. Marie Walsh, Laguna Hills, California, Winter 1992.
79. Statistics released by Susan Cruzan of the FDA Press Office, personal communication, May 1993.
80. 1992 FDA Panel Review transcript, note 1, pp. 349-351 (Day 1).
81. transcript, note 1, p. 204 (Day 2).

## *Chapter Seven: The Aftermath*

1. Elinor Breher, "An explanation of FDA panel's recommendation on implants," *Miami Herald*, 1 March 1992, sec. J, p. 5.
2. 1992 FDA Panel transcript, Ch. six, note 1, pp. 200 and 210 (Day 3).
3. transcript, p. 390 (Day 2).
4. transcript, pp. 412-413 (Day 2).
5. transcript, p. 187 (Day 1).
6. "Update on silicone gel-filled breast implants," U. S. Department of Health and Human Services, Food and Drug Administration (FDA), Rockville, Maryland 20857, 27 May 1992.
7. *HHS News*, U. S. Department of Health and Human Services, note 6, 11 April 1992.
8. "Update on silicone gel-filled breast implants," note 6.
9. Letter from George Gerstenburg, District Director, Los Angeles District Office, FDA, to Donald K. McGhan, CEO and Chairman of the Board, McGhan Medical Corporation, dated 31 March 1992; reported in "The FDA's regulation of silicone breast implants," a December 1992 staff report by the Human Resources and Intergovernmental Relations Subcommittee of the Committee on Government Operations (Washington, D.C.: U. S. Government Printing Office, 1993), p. 42.
10. Press release from the Office of Consumer Affairs, authorizing an exemption for the implantation of McGhan's style 153 Biocell Anatomical Reconstructive Silicone gel-filled Breast Implant. Reported in *B. I. F. F. Newsletter*, Ch. 6, note 78, fall 1992.
11. "The FDA's regulation of silicone gel implants," note 9, pp. 46-47.
12. The Human Resources and Intergovernmental Relations Subcommittee's findings were cited in "Report: U.S. lax on retin-a and silicone," *Orange County Register*, 23 November 1992.
13. *HHS News*, note 7.

14. John Schwartz, "Study finds no link to disease," *Washington Post*, 16 June 1994, sec. A, p. 1.
15. 1992 FDA Panel Review transcript, Ch. 6, note 1, p. 16 (Day 2).
16. *Federal Register*, Ch. 4, note 25.
17. The document was received by the FDA advisory committee members prior to the 13-14 November 1988 Panel Review; cited in "The FDA's regulation of silicone breast implants," note 9, p. 7.
18. "Update on slicone gel-filled breast implants," note 6, p. 7.
19. Susan Blakeslee (*New York Times*), "Doctor, carcinogen found in mom who has implants," *Orange County Register*, 2 June 1991; Nicholas Regush, "Toxic Breasts," *Mother Jones*, January/February 1992.
20. "The FDA's regulation of silicone breast implants," note 9, p. 35.
21. "Investigative report criticizes FDA's failure to regulate breast implants," 7 January 1992 Press Release by Congressman Donald Payne, 10th district, New Jersey, summarizing the three year investigation of the FDA by the Human Resouces and Intergovernmental Relations Subcommittee of the House Committee on Government Operations; subcommittee report, note 9.
22. "The FDA's regulation of silicone breast implants," note 9, p. 37.
23. "The FDA's regulation of silicone breast implants," pp. 37-38.
24. Marc Lappe, *Chemical Deceptions* (San Fransisco: Sierra Club Books, 1991); see also Ch. 9; Ch. 5.
25. "The FDA's regulation of silicone breast implants," note 9, p. 40.
26. "The FDA's regulation of silicone breast implants," p. 44.
27. Rep. Payne, note 20.
28. D. de Camera, J. M. Sheridan, B. A. Kramer, "Rupture and aging of silicone breast implants," presented at the 1991 annual meeting of the ASPRS; reported in *USA Today*, September 1991; see also FDA Panel Review transcript, Ch. 6, note 1, p. 147 (Day 1).
29. 1992 FDA Panel Review transcript, pp. 535 and 538 (Day 2).
30. transcript, pp. 145 and 188 (Day 1).
31. transcript, p. 115 (Day 1).
32. transcript, p. 124 (Day 1); see also: I. K. Cohen and M. Scheflan, "The value of xeromammography for ruptured breast implants," [letter] *Plastic and Reconstructive Surgery*, 69 (1982), 898-900; I. K. Cohen et al., "Xeromammography: a reason for using saline-filled breast prostheses." *Plastic and Reconstructive Surgery*, 60 (1977), 886-88.

33. Jeff Fitzsimmons and B. Steinbach preliminary report published in *Investigation Radiology,* October (1992). See also R. F. Brem, C. M. Tempany, and E.A. Zerhouni, "MR detection of breast implant rupture," *Journal of Computer Assisted Tomography,* 16 (1) (1992), 157-9.

34. 1992 FDA Panel Review transcript, Ch. 6, note 1, pp. 334-35 (Day 2).

35. transcript, p. 415 (Day 2).

36. transcript, p. 405 (Day 2).

37. transcript, p. 408 (Day 2).

38. Nancy Brunning, *Breast Implants, Everything You Want to Know* (Alameda, California: Hunter House, 1992), p. 75.

39. 1992 FDA Panel Review transcript, Ch. 6, note 1 p. 493 (Day 2).

40. The proposal was presented to a Consumer Briefing Meeting, Washington, D.C. on 9 June 1992. To object to this proposal contact: PHS Implant Task Force, National Institute of Health, Bethesda, Maryland, 20815.

41. Personal communication, March 1993.

42. 1992 FDA Panel Review transcript, Ch. 6, note 1, p. 496 (Day 2).

43. Thomas M. Burton, "Breast implants raise more safety issues," (part 1) "Research links silicone version to new disease," and Joan E. Rigdon, "Breast implants raise more safety issues," (part 2) "Saline implants appear to carry safety hazards as well," *Wall Street Journal,* 4 February 1993.

44. Jane Harper, "Houston surgeons sue over silicone implants," *Houston Post,* 16 February 1993, sec. A, p. 1.

45. *B. I. F. F. Newsletter,* Ch. 6, note 78, June 1993, vol. 17, p. 4.

46. Statistics released by Susan Cruzan of the FDA Press Office, personal communication, 6 May 1993.

47. The Associated Press, "Lawsuit says penile implants dangerous," Ft. Lauderdale *Sun Sentinel,* 21 May 1994, sec. A, p. 15.

48. The Associated Press, "Lawsuit says penile implants dangerous," Ft. Lauderdale *Sun Sentinel,* 21 May 1994, sec. A. p.15

### *Chapter Eight: Other Devices, Other Dangers*

1.  1992 FDA Panel Review transcript, Ch. 6, note 1, pp. 158-159 (Day 1)

.2. "The FDA's regulation of silicone breast implants," p. 3; Dow Corning filed the Notice of Claimed Investigational Exemption for a New Drug (IND) in 1965.

3.  "FDA's regulation of silicone breast implants," note 9, p. 3; see also Ch. 4, note 16.

4. Tony Randall, "Less maligned, but cut from the same cloth, other silicone implants also have adverse effects," *Journal of the American Medical Association*, 268 (1) (1992), 12-13.

5. Susan Blakeslee, "Data suggest that implants may pose risk of later harm," *New York Times*, 25 July 1989, sec. C, p. 1.

6. Randall, note 4; lipid infiltration as a contributory factor, see R. Van Moor, M. M. Black, and B. Harris, "Developments in the biomedical evaluation of silicone rubber," *Journal of Materials in Science*, 14 (1979), 197.

7. Lappe, note 23.

8. Caroline Acton et al., "Silicone-induced foreign body reaction after temporomandibular joint arthroplasty: case report," *Australian Dental Journal*, 34 (3) (1989), 288-232; J. M. Barrett, D. C. O'Sullivan, A. A. Malizia, et al., "Particle shedding and migration from silicone genitourinary prosthetic devices," *Journal of Urology*, 146 (July-August) (1991), 319-22; Franklin Dolwick and Thomas B. Aufdemort, "Silicone-induced foreign body and lymphadenopathy after temporomandibular joint arthroplasty," *Oral Surgery, Oral Medicine, Oral Pathology*, 59 (1985), 449-452; Michael Gordon and Peter G. Bullough, "Synovial and osseous inflammation in failed silicone-rubber prostheses: a report of six cases," *Journal of Bone and Joint Surgery*, 64-A (4) (1982), 574-580; Gerald D. Groff, Alan K. Scned, and Thomas H. Taylor, "Silicone-induced adenopathy eight years after metacarpophalangeal arthroplasty," *Arthritis and Rheumatism*, 24 (December) (1981), 1578-1581; M. A. Lazaro, D. G. Morteo, and M. A. Benyacar, "Lymphadenopathy secondary to silicone hand joint prostheses." *Clinical Experimental Rheumatology*, 8 (1) (1950), 17-22; Clayton Peimer, John Medige, Barry S. Eckect, et al., "Reactive Synovitis after silicone arthroplasty," *Journal of Hand Surgery*, 11-A (5) (1986), 624-638; S. H. Paplanus and C. M. Payne, "Auxillary Lymphaenopathy 17 years after digitial silicone implants: study with x-ray microanalysis," *Journal of Hand Surgery*, 13-A (1988), 411-12; Daniel I. Rosenthal et al., "Destructive arthritis due to silicone: a foreign body rection," *Radiology*, 149 (October) (1983), 69-72; Robert A. Worsing et al., "Reactive Synovitis from particulate silastic," *Journal of Bone and Joint Surgery*, 64-A (April) (1982), 581-585; P. L. Westesson et al., "Destructive lesions of the mandibular condyle following diskectomy with silicone implants," *Oral Surgery, Oral Medicine, Oral Pathology*, 63 (2) (1987), 143-49.

9. Dolwick and Aufdemort, note 8; A. J. Christie, K. A. Weinburger, and M. Dietriech, "Silicone lymphadenopathy and Synovitis complications of silicone elastomer finger joint prostheses," *Journal of the American Medical Association,* 37 (2) (1977), 1463-64; Gordon and Bullough; Groff, Scned, and Taylor, note 8; T. Kircher, "Silicone lyphadenopathy: a complication of silicone elastomer finger joint prostheses," *Human Pathology,* 11 (1980), 240-244; Randall, note 4; Rosenthal et al., Westesson et al., Worsing et al., note 8.

10. Barnett, O'Sullivan, Malizza, et al., note 8; Randall, note 4.

11. Silver, Ch. 6, note 59. References: Christie, Weinburg, and Dietriech, note 8; Lazaro, Morteo, and de Benyacar; Paplanus and Payne, note 8.

12. Robert G. Apetar, Joseph M. Davie, and Hereward S. Cattell, "Foreign body reaction to silicone rubber. Complications of a finger joint implant," *Clinical Orthopaedics and Related Research,* 98 (1974), 231-32; Christie, Weinburger, and Dietriech, note 9; D. C. Ferlic, M. L. Claylon, and M. Halloway, "Complications of silicone implant surgery in the metacarpophalangeal joint," *Journal of Bone and Joint Surgery,* 57-A (1975), 991-94; Gordon and Bullough, note 8; Kircher, note 8; Peimer, Medige, Eckert, et al., note 68; Rosenthal et al., note 68; Worsing et al., note 68.

13. Tony Randall, "Surgeons grapple with Synovitis, fractures around silicone implants for hand and wrist," *Journal of the American Medical Association,* 268 (1) (1992), 13-18.

14. Peimer, Medige, Eckert, et al., note 8.

15. Randall, note 13.

16. Food and Drug Administration, *Federal Register* 55 no. 96, 17 May 1990, p. 20571.

17. The estimate of Dr. Alfred B. Swanson, inventor of silicone finger and wrist implants, cited in Randall, note 13.

18. Dolwick and Aufdemort, note 8.

19. Wanda Woo, "Lawsuits over jaw implants proliferate," *Wall Street Journal,* 11 May 1993.

20. Attorney Harriet Lewis of Hollywood, Florida; personal communication, 6 May 1992.

21. Woo, note 19.

22. Philip J. Hilts, "Strange history of silicone held many warnings," *New York Times,* 18 January 1992; see also note 23.

23. N. Valentin and R. Vilhelmsen, "Blood and tissue silicon in extracorporeal circulation," *Journal of Cardiovascular Surgery,* 17

(January) (1976), 20-26; see also D. A. B. Lindberg, F. V. Lucas, J. Sheagren, et al., "Silicone embolization during clinical and experimental heart surgery employing a bubble oxygenator," *American Journal of Pathology*, 39 (1961), 129; Jan Marc Orenstein, Noriko Sato, Benjamin Aaron, et al., "Microemboli observed in deaths following cardiopulmonary bypass surgery: silicone antifoam agents and polyvinyl chloride tubing as sources of emboli," *Human Pathology*, 13 (1982), 1082-90; Robert W. Thomassen et al., "The occurrence and characterization of emboli associated with the use of a silicone antifoam agent," *Journal of Thoracic Cardiovascular Surgery*, 41 (1961), 611-22.

24. Michael Merle, A. Lee Dellon, James N. Campbell, and Peter S. Chang, "Complications from silicon-polymer intubation of nerves," *Microsurgery*, 10 (1989), 130-33.

25. William D. Travis, Karoly Balogh, Barbara C. Wolfe, et al., "Silicone-induced endocarditis," *Archives of Pathology and Laboratory Medicine*, 110 (January) (1986), 51-54.

26. J. Hunt and M J. G. Farthing, "Silicone in the liver: possible late effects," *Gut*, 30 (2) (1989), 239-42; see also note 27.

27. Hilts, note 22; see also Nir Kossovsky, P. Cole, and D. A. Jackson, "Giant cell myocarditis associated with silicone. An unusual case discovered at autopsy using x-ray energy spectroscopic techniques," *Journal of Clinical Pathology*, 93 (11) (1990), 148-52; A. S. Y. Leong, A. P. S. Disney, and D. W. Grove, "Spallation and migration of silicone from blood-pumping tubing in patients on haemodialysis," *New England Journal of Medicine*, 306 (1982), 135; A. S. Y. Leong, A. P. S. Disney, and D. W. Grove, [letter to the editor] "Refractive particles in liver of haemodialysis patients," *Lancet*, (April 18) (1981), 889; P. S. Parfray, J. B. O'Driscoll, and F. J. Paradinas, "Refractive material in the liver of haemodialysis patients," *Lancet*, 1 (1981), 1101; C. F. W. Wolf, "Hepatic silicone emboli due to fragmentation of roller pump tubing," *International Journal of Artificial Organs*, 5 (1982), 277.

28. See notes7 and 8.

29. Laura Campbell, "Wright looks at new tools, new day," *Memphis Commercial Appeal*, 20 June 1993, sec. C, p. 1.

30. Abbie Jones, "Implant impact: European health officials question U. S. Ban," *Today's Boca Woman*, Boca Raton, Florida, September 1992, pp. 17-19.

31. R. I. Press, C. L. Peebles, Y. Kumagai, R. L. Ochs, and E. Tan, "Antinuclear antibodies in women with silicone breast implants," *Lancet*,

340 (November) (1992), 1304-07; see also Palm Beach Wire Service, "Implant injuries linked to disease," *Palm Beach Post,* 28 November 1992.

32. David A. Kessler, R. B. Merkatz, and R. Schapino, "A call for higher standards for breast implants," *Journal of the American Medical Association,* 270 (no. 21) (December) (1993), 2607-2608.

33. Council in Scientific Affairs, American Medical Association, "Silicone gel breast implants," *Journal of the American Medical Association,* 270 (no. 21) (December) (1993), 2602-2606.

## Chapter Nine: An Appraisal of Risks

1. Sidney M. Wolfe, *Women's Health Alert* (Reading, Massachusetts: Addison-Wesley Publishing Company, Inc., 1990), p. 22.

2. C. Rolland, R. Guidoin, D. Marceau, and R. Ledoux, "Nondestructive investigations on ninety-six surgically excised mammary prostheses," *Journal of Biomedical Materials Research,* 23 (A3 supplement) (December) (1989), 285-98.

3. Dr. Britta Ostermeyer-Shoaib of Baylor College of Medicine, Houston; presentation: State of Florida Silicone Seminar, Tampa, Florida, 23 January 1993.

4. "Some problems after breast implant surgery reported to the network: we have not seen these in the medical literature," *CTN Newsletter,* Ch. 6, note 26, Winter 1989-90.

5. W. M. Cocke Jr. and H. W. Sampson, "Silicone bleed associated with double-lumen breast prostheses," *Annals of Plastic Surgery,* 18 (1987), 524-26.

6. Atel Vargas, "Shedding of silicone particles from inflated breast implants," [letter] *Plastic and Reconstructive Surgery,* 64 (1974), 252-53; see also Ch. 8, pp. 174-177, notes 7-17.

7. Lappe, Ch. 7, note 23.

8. Janet Van Winkle, Founder of American Silicone Survivors, "Prepared statement before the Part 15 Hearing: Saline Breast Implants," Washington, D.C., 2 June 1994, p. 3.

9. Britta Ostermeyer-Shoaib and Bernard M. Patten, "Rheumatologic and neurologic findings in silicone adjuvant breast disease," in *CTN Newsletter,* Ch. 6, note 26, 7 November 1992; see also note 11.

10. Dr. Frank Vasey, during: The State of Florida Silicone Seminar, note 3.

11. N. A. Fenske and Frank B. Vasey, "Silicone-associated connective-tissue disease," *Archives of Dermatology,* 129 January (1993), 97-98. Reference: L. A. Love, Steven R. Weiner, Frank B. Vasey, et al., "Clinical

immunogenic features of women who develop myositis after silicone implants (MASI)," *Arthritis and Rheumatism*, 35 (1992), S46; see also Vasey, Bocanegra, Havice, et a., Ch. 6, note 69.

12. Alan J. Bridges, Carol Conley, Grace Wang, David E. Burns, and Frank B. Vasey, "A clinical immunological evaluation of women with silicone breast implants and symptoms of rheumatic disease," *Arthritis and Rheumatism*, 35 (1992), S65.

13. S. A. Tenebaum, L. H. Silveira, B. Martinez-Osuna, M. L. Cuellar, R. F. Garry, and L. R. Espinoza, "Identification of a novel auto-antigen recognized in silicone-associated disease," *Artritis and Rheumatism*, 35 (12) (1992), S73; cited in Fenske and Vasey, note 11.

14. "Immunology studies on silicone gel" in *FDA Talk Paper* (T93-15), U. S. Department of Health and Human Services, Rockville, Maryland, 23 March 1993.

15. J. O. Naim, R. J. Lanzafame, and C. T. Van Oss, "The adjuvant effect of silicone-gel on antibody formation in rats," Immunological Investigation, 22 (1993), 151-161.

16. Food and Drug Administration, "Breast implants, a consumer information update," June 1993, p. 2.

17. C. Petit (San Francisco Chronicle), "Illnesses linked to implants," *The Orange County Register*, 15 March 1993, sec. A, p. 3; see also *B. I. F. F. Newsletter*, Ch. 6, note 78, vol. 17, p. 4.

18. Published in *B. I. F. F. Newsletter*, Ch. 6, note 78, July 1993, vol. 18, p. 5. (Attorneys plan to enter the cited study in court during the next breast implant liability trial.)

19. See Ch. 4, note 6.

20. FDA 515B Regulation Preamble, 1989 draft, cited in Sidney M. Wolfe, *Women's Health Alert*, note 1, p. 26.

21. See note 3.

22. New York Times News Service, "Researchers probing mystery of chronic fatigue syndrome," *The Palm Beach Post*, 20 January 1993, sec. D, p. 9.

23. *The Palm Beach Post*, 20 Jaunuary 1993, sec. D., p. 9.

24. 1992 FDA Panel Review transcript, Ch. 6, note 1, p. 221 (Day 2).

25. "Immunomediator cytokines secreted in capsules," a paper presented to the American College of Rheumatology, 11 September 1993, San Antonio, Texas; reported in a 21 October 1993 letter to the Multidistrict Litigation (MDL) Plaintiffs Steering Committee from attorney Aaron M. Levine, Science and Causation Committee, Washington, D.C.,

26. 1992 FDA Panel Review transcript, Ch. 6, note 1, p. 350 (Day 1); see also note 25.
27. Ostermeyer-Shoaib, note 3.
28. J. R. Sanger, H. S. Matloub, N. J. Yousif, and R. Komorowski, "Silicone gel infiltration of a peripheral nerve and constrictive neuropathy following rupture of a breast prosthesis," *Plastic and Reconstructive Surgery,* 89 May (1992), 949-52.
29. Dr. Britta Ostermeyer-Shoaib, Baylor College of Medicine, Houston, personal communication, March 1993; see also 1992 FDA Panel Review transcript, Ch. 6, note 1, p. 250 (Day 1).
30. 1992 FDA Panel Review transcript, Ch. 6, note 1, pp. 542-47 (Day 2); see also Patten, transcript, pp. 251, 362 (Day 1).
31. T. A. Fassel, J. E. Van Over, C. C. Hausner, C. E. Edminston, and J. R. Sanger, "Adhesion of staphylococci to breast implant prosthesis biomaterials: an electron microscope evaluation," *Cells and Materials,* 1 (3) (1991), 199-08; Thomas J. Krizek, "The normal body defenses against foreign implants," in *Biomaterials in Reconstructive Surgery,* ed. Leonard R. Rubin (St. Loius: C. V. Mosby Company, 1983), pp. 9-15; C. Rolland, R. Ledoux, R. Guidoin, et al., "First observations of hopeite and parascholzite in fibrous capsules surrounding silicone breast implants," *International Journal of Artificial Organs,* 12 March (1989), 180-08; C. Rolland, R. Guidoin, R. Ledoux, et al., "Carbonate-hydroxylapatite, hopeite, and parascholzite in fibrous capsule surrounding breast implants," *Canada Minerologist,* 29 (2) (1991), 337-45; J. R. Sanger, N. K. Sheth, and T. R. Franson, "Adherence of microorganisms to breast prostheses: an in vitro study," *Annals of Plastic Surgery,* 22 (April) (1989), 337-42; D. Sanyal and C. Thurston, "Mycoplasma hominis infection of a breast prosthesis," [letter] *Journal of Infection,* 23 (2) (September) (1991), 210-11; C. Umansky, "Infections with polyurethane-coated implants," [correspondence] *Plastic and Reconstructive Surgery,* 75 (1985), 925-26.
32. D. E. Berman, J. Lettieri, et al., "Steroid and benzyl alcohol diffusion through tissue expanders and double lumen breast implants," *Annals of Plastic Surgery,* 27 (4) (October) (1991), 316-20; B. R. Burkhardt et al., "Capsular contracture: a prospective study of the effect of local antibacterial agents," *Plastic and Reconstructive Surgery,* 77 (1986), 919-30; B. R. Burkhardt et al., "Capsules, infection, and intraluminal antibiotics," *Plastic and Reconstructive Surgery,* 68 (1981), 43; T. J. Carrico and I. K. Cohen, "Capsular contracture and steroid related complications after augmentation mammaplasty," *Plastic and Reconstructive Surgery,* 64

March (1979), 337-80; C. W. D. Morain, "The role of iodine-releasing silicone implants in the prevention of spherical contracture in mice," [Discussion] *Plastic and Reconstructive Surgery*, 69 (1982), 960; R. O'Neal and L. Argenta, "Late side effects related to inflatable breast prostheses containing soluble steroids," *Plastic and Reconstructive Surgery*, 66 (1980), 71-73; E. R. Perrin, "The use of soluble steroids in inflatable breast prostheses," *Plastic and Reconstructive Surgery*, 57 (1976), 163; S. L. Spear, H. Matsuba, S. Romm, and J. W. Little, "Methyl prednisone in double-lumen gel-saline submuscular mammary prostheses: a double-blind, prospective, controlled clinical trial," *Plastic and Reconstructive Surgery*, 87 (March) (1991), 483-87, and discussion, 488-89; K. Weinbren, R. Salm, and G. Greenberg, "Intramuscular injections of iron compounds and oncogenesis in men," *British Medical Journal*, 1 (1978), 683-85.

33. D.E. Berman, J. Lettieri, et al., "Steroid and Benzyl alcohol diffusion through tissue expanders and double lumen breast implants," *Annals of Plastic Surgery*, 27 (4) (October) (1991), p. 316-20.

34. 1992 FDA Panel Review transcript, Ch. 6, note 1, pp. 116-26 (Day 1); see also "Bracing for the tide of augmentation-breast films," *Physician Weekly*, 12 June 1989; H. Hayes Jr., J. Vandergrift, and W. C. Diner, "Mammography and breast implants," *Plastic and Reconstructive Surgery*, 82 (1) (1988), 1-88; S. H. Heywang, E. Eiermann, R. Basserman, et al., "Carcinoma of the breast behind a prosthesis - comparison of ultrasound, mammography, and MRI (case report)," *Computerized Radiology*, 9 (1985), 283-86; Melvin J. Silverstein, "Augmentation mammaplasty - its effects on breast cancer diagnosis and prognosis," *Archives of Surgery*, 123 (June) (1988), 681-85; Melvin J. Silverstein, P. Gamagami, and N. Handel, "Missed breast cancer in an augmented women using implant displacement mammography," *Annals of Plastic Surgery*, 25 (3) (September) (1990), 210-13; J. N. Wolfe, "On mammography in the presence of breast implants," [a letter to the editor] *Plastic and Reconstructive Surgery*, 62 (1978), 286; Sidney M. Wolfe, note 1. p. 24.

35. Melvin J. Silverstein, E. D. Gierson, P. Gamagami, et al., "Breast cancer diagnosis in women with silicone gel-filled implants," *Cancer*, 66 (July 1) (1990), 97-101; Silverstein, Gamagami, and Handel, note 34. Silverstein, note 35; see also Melvin J. Silverstein, N. Handel, and P. Gamagami, "The effects of silicone gel-filled implants and mammography," *Cancer*, 68 (September) 1 (1991), 1159-63; Melvin J. Silverstein, G. P. Murphy, J.

Bostwick, et al., "Breast reconstruction. State of the art for the 1990's," *Cancer,* 68 (September 1) (1991), 1180-81.

36. Susan M. Love, *Dr. Love's Breast Book,* (Reading, Massachusetts: Addison-Wesley Publishing Company, Inc., 1990), pp. 137-43.

37. Wolfe, note 1, p. 24.

38. Hayes, Vandergrift, and Diner, note 34; R. T. Schmidt, G. N. Peters, and W. P. Evans, "Silicone implants and breast cancer: another prospective," *Proceedings of the Annual Meeting of the American Society of Clinical Oncology,* 7 (1988), A88; Silverstein et al., note 34; Silverstein, Gierson, Gamagami, et al.; Silverstein, Handel, and Gamagami, note 35.

39. Public Citizen Health Research Group (PCHRG) *Health Letter,* December 1988, vol. 4, no. 12; see also T. Wirth, "[The effect of asbestos cement, UICC asbestos samples and quartz on the peritoneum of the mouse]," [German] *Pathologia et Microbiologia,* 42 (1) (1975), 15-28.

40. Habal, Ch. 2, note 2.

41. Reference to silicone's containment of peroxides, platinum, and solid or fumed silica: R. Gayou and R. Rudolph, "Capsular contracture around silicone mammary prostheses," *Annals of Plastic Surgery,* 2 (1) (1979), 62-71; see also Haley; Redinger Van Aken et al; ard, Ch. 4, note 26.

42. Lappe, Ch. 7, note 23, p. 155. References: S. L. Robbins, R. S. Cottran, and V. Kumar, *Pathological Basis of Disease,* 3rd ed. (Philadelphia: Sanders, 1984), pp. 435-37; M. P. Absher et al., "Biphasic cellular and tissue response to rat lungs after eight-day aerosal exposure to silicon dioxide cristobabite," *American Journal of Pathology,* 134 (1989), 1243-47.

43. S. C. Chan, D. C. Birdsell, and C. Y. Gradeen, "Detection of toluenediamines in the urine of a patient with polyurethane-covered breast implants," *Clinical Chemistry,* 37 (5) (1991), 756-58; S. C. Chan, D. C. Birdsell, and C. Y. Gradeen, "Urinary excretion of free toluenediamines in the urine of a patient with polyurethane-covered breast implants," *Clinical Chemistry,* 37 (12) (1991), 2143-45; New York Times News Service, "Silicone breasts leak chemical, test shows," *The Commerical Appeal,* 25 September 1993, sec. A, p. 4; see also Susan Blakeslee (*New York Times*), "Doctor: carcinogen found in milk of mom who has implants," *Orange County Register,* 2 June 1991.

44. "Breast Implant Award," *The National Law Journal,* 25 March 1991; E. Frost, "Breast implant cancer link alleged," *ABA Journal,* June 1991, p. 18; Carla Rohlfing, "Is there a time bomb ticking in women's chests," *Longevity,* July 1991.

45. Noted in the technical data sheet (TDS) on the manufacturing process; reported at the Association of Trial Lawyers of America (ATLA) Breast Implant Group Litigation Seminar, Ch. 4, note 19. Summary memorandum dated 23 January 1992, item 57.

46. Reuters, "$25 million awarded in Texas implants case," *Palm Beach Post*, 24 December 1992.

47. Lappe, Ch. 7, note 23, p. 98.

48. Food and Drug Administration, *Federal Register* (21 CFR part 878) 55 (96), 17 May 1990, p. 20571. References: J. Autian, "Toxicological aspects of implants," *Journal of Biomaterials Research*, 1 (1967), 433; J. Autian et al., "Carcinogenesis from polyurethane," *Cancer Research*, 35 (1975), 1591-96; N. Ben-Hur and Z. Neuman, "Malignant tumor formation following subcutaneous injection of silicone fluid in white mice," *Israel Medical Journal*, 22 (1963), 15; W. C. Hueper, "Cancer induction by polyurethane and polysilicone plastics," *Journal of the National Cancer Institute*, 33 (1964), 1005-27; W. C. Hueper, "Experimental production of cancer by means of implanted polyurethane plastic," *American Journal of Clinical Pathology*, 34 (1960), 328-33; R. B. Pedley, G. Meachim, and D. F. Williams, "Tumor induction by implant materials," in "Fundamental Aspects of Biocompatibility," *CRC Critical Reviews in Biocompatibility*, ed. D. F. Williams (Boca Raton, Florida: CRC Press, 1981), vol. II, 175-202.

49. A summary of medical literature prepared by FDA staff entitled: "Risk and benefits of silicone gel-filled breast implants, a summary of findings in the literature," provided in the information packet of the support group B. I. F. F. (Breast Implant Information Foundation), Laguna Hills, California. The FDA received the Dow Corning 2 year (1985-87) rat bioassays of MDF-0193 and 97 2159A silicone gels (fibrosarcoma findings) in March of 1988. During a 26 January 1989 General and Plastic Surgery Devices Panel Meeting, Dr. Mishra of the FDA discussed an FDA letter written to Dow Corning in request of "all test data on silicone breast implants." At that time, a company representative acknowledged the FDA's receipt of a summarized list of 750 biosafety studies, 39 toxicology studies, and a completed report on the 2 year (1976-78) Industrial Biotest Labs Study (lymphoma findings). Summaries of FDA transcripts of General and Plastic Surgery Devices Panel Meetings, Ch. 5, note 2.

50. Sheridan, "Review of toxicity data for silicone gels," Ch. 5, note 17.

51. Luu, "Master file silicone Dow Corning," Ch. 5, note 20.

52. Dennis M. Deapen, Malcolm C. Pike, John T. Casagrande, et al., "The relationship between breast cancer and augmentation mammaplasty: an epidemiologic study," *Plastic and Reconstructive Surgery*, 77 (1986), 361-65.

53. Dr. Sidney M. Wolfe, Director of PCHRG, quoted the 25 July 1988 internal FDA review of the Deapen study during testimony (PCHRG publication #1149) before the 22 November 198 FDA Advisory Committee on General and Plastic Surgery Devices.

54. Lynn Rosenberg, "The relationship between breast cancer and augmentation mammaplasty: an epidemiologic study," *Plastic and Reconstructive Surgery*, 77 (1986), 368.

55. J. Autian, "The new field of plastics toxicology: methods and results," *CRC Critical Reviews on Toxicology*, 2 (1973), 1; see also Autian, Autian et al., and Hueper, note 47.

56. Reported at the Assocation of Trial Lawyers of America (ATLA) Breast Implant Litigation Group Seminar, Ch. 4, note 14. Summary memorandum dated 23 January 1992, item 57; see also Ch. 5, note 20, and Ch.4, note 14.

57. Tim M. Smart, "Breast implants: What did the industry know and when?" *Business Week*, 10 June 1991, pp. 94-98.

58. F. Bishoff and G. Bryson, "Carcinogenesis through solid state surfaces," *Progress in Experimental Tumor Research*, 5 (1964), 85; F. Bishoff, "Carcinogenic effect of steroids," *Advances in Lipid Research*, 7 (1969), 165.

59. Lappe, Ch. 7, note 23, p. 169.

60. Lappe. Reference: M. Holloway, "A great poison," *Scientific American*, 263 (1990), 16-20.

61. 1992 FDA Panel Review transcript, Ch. 6, note 1, p. 378 (Day 1).

62. Love, note 36, p. 144.

63. Love. Reference: A. T. McMahon, P. Cole, and J. Brown, "Etiology of human breast cancer: a review," *Journal of the National Cancer Institute*, 50 (1973), 21-42.

64. Lappe, Ch. 7, note 23, p. 177. Reference: M. S. Berstein, R. L. Hunter, and S. Yachnin, "Hematomas and oral contraceptives," *Lancet*, 2 (1971), 1273-76.

65. Lappe, Ch. 7, note 23, p. 175. Reference: L. Plapinger and H. A. Bern, "Adenosis-like lesions and other cervicovaginal abnormalities in mice treated neonatally with estrogen," *Journal of the National Cancer Institute*, 64 (1979), 507-18.

66. Lappe, p. 176. Reference: W. S. Branham et al., "Alterations in developing rat uterine cell populations after neonatal exposure to estrogens and antiestrogens," *Teratology*, 38 (1988), 271-279.

67. J. H. Hartley Jr. and William F. Schatten, "Postoperative complications of lactation after mammaplasty," *Plastic and Reconstructive Surgery*, 47 (2) (1971), 150-53; Mary H. McGrath and Boyd R. Burhardt, "The safety and efficacy of breast implants for augmentation mammaplasty," *Plastic and Reconstructive Surgery*, 74 (4) (1984), 550-60; see also T. C. Mason, "Hyperprolactinemia and galactorrhea associated with mammary prostheses and unresponsive to bromocriptine. A case report," *Journal of Reproductive Medicine*, 36 (A) (1991), 541-42.

68. Lappe, Ch. 7, note 23, pp. 125-26.

69. Lappe, pp. 132-33.

70. Lappe, p. 126.

71. Lappe, p. 98.

72. Lappe, p. 126.

73. Lappe, pp. 148 and 162. Reference: S. M. Barlow and A. M. Knight, "Teratogenic effects of silastic intrauterine devices in the rat with or without added medroxyprogesterone," *Fertility and Sterility*, 39 (1983), 224-30.

74. H. Bates, R. Filler, and C. Kimmel, "Development toxicity study of polydimethylsiloxane injection in the rat," *Teratology*, 31 (1985), 50A.

50. G. L. Kennedy, M. L. Keplinger, J. C. Calandra, and E. J. Hobbs, "Reproductive, teratologic and mutagenic studies with some polydimethylsiloxanes," *Journal of Toxicology and Environmental Health*, 1 (1976), 909-20; see also Barlow and Knight, note 73; McGrath and Burkhardt, note 67.

75. "Some problems after breast implant surgery reported to the network: we have not seen these in the literature," note 4.

76. Data collected by the C.A.T.S. (Children Afflicted by Toxic Substances) Northport, New York; distributed by Command Trust Network (CTN), Covington, Kentucky.

77. Thomas M. Burton, "Breast implants raise more safety issues," (Part I) "Resarch links silicone version to new diseases," *Wall Street Journal*, 4 February 1993, sec. B, p. 1.

78. Marianne Neifert, Sandra De Manzo, Joy Seacat, et al., "The influence of breast surgery, breast appearance, and pregnancy-induced breast changes on lactation sufficency as measured by infant weight gain," (A prosective study funded by NICHS) *Birth*, 17 91) (1990), 31-39; see also *Lactation:*

# TORN ILLUSIONS

*Phsiology, Nutrition, and Breast Feeding,* ed. Margaret C. Neville and Marianne Neifert (New York: Plenum Press, 1983), pp. 343-44.

79. Ostemeyer-Shoaib, note 3.
80. Nancy McVicar, "Breast-feeding with implants linked to problems," Ft. Lauderdale *Sun Sentinel,* 19 January 1994, sec. A, p. 11; see Jeremiah J. Levine and Norman T. Llowite, "Sclerodermalike esophageal disease in children breast-fed by mothers with silicone breast implants," *Journal of the American Medical Association,* 271 (January 19) (3) (1994), 213-216
81. Reported in *B. I. F. F. Newsletter,* Ch. 6, note 79, vol. 14, Winter 1992.

## *Chapter 10: The Victims*

1. Michael Castleman, "Women's Warrior," *California Lawyer,* March 1993, pp. 45-105.
2. Leslie Bryan of Doffernyre, Shields, Canfield, and Knowles, Atlanta, Georgia, personal communication, 6 May 1993. (Attorney Frank Knowles is Co-Chair of the MDL Plaintiff Steering Committee.)
3. Transcript: 24 February 1992 Silicone Breast Implant Hearing, United States District Court, Northern District of Alabama, South Division, re: Silicone gel breast implants no. CV 92-P-10000-S, products liability litigation (MDL-926), San Francisco, California.
4. Transcript: 24 February 1992 Silicone Breast Implant Hearing; see also James P. Miller, "Dow Corning says grand jury studies firm's handling of breast-implant data," *Wall Street Journal,* 18 February 1993.
5. Thomas M. Burton, "Dow Corning refuses to give the FDA independent report on breast implants," *Wall Street Journal,* 15 January 1993.
6. Burton.
7. Reported in *C. O. S. S. Newsletter,* (Coalition of Silicone Survivors), ed. Lynda Roth, Broomfiled, Colorado June 1993.
8. "Global settlement negotiations conducted in secret," *Mealey's Litigation Report,* ed. Mealey's Publications, Wayne, Pensylvania, 8 April 1993.
9. Reported in the *Multidistrict Breast Implant Litigation Reporter,* ed. MDL Plaintiff Steering Committee, vol. 1 no. 5, March-April 1993, p. 5.
10. Gina Kolata, "Fund proposed for settling suits over breast implants," *The New York Times,* 9 September 1994, sec. A, p. 11.
11. "Statement of Principles for Global Resolution of Implant Claims," dated 3 September 1993, provided by Leslie J. Bryan, office of Doffernyre, Shields, Canfield, and Knowles, Atlanta, Georgia.

12. 23 September 1993 letter from Dr. Norman Anderson, John Hopkins School of Medicine, Baltimore, Maryland, to attorney Dan Bolton of Wilson, Szumowski, and Bolton, San Francisco, California.

13. 13 September 1993 letter from MDL Plaintiff Steering Committee member Dan Bolton, of Wilson, Szumowski, and Bolton, San Francisco, CA., to the MDL Plaintiff Steering Committee and the Advisory Committee; provided by *C. O. S. S. Newsletter,* October 1993.

14. 27 September 1993 letter from attorney Christopher M. Placitella of Wilentz, Goldman, and Spitzer, Woodbridge, New Jersey, to the Honorable C. Judson Hamlin, Middlesex County Supreme Court, New Brunswick, New Jersey; provided by the National Breast Implant Plaintiffs' Coalition, note 16.

15. 21 October 1993 letter from Gail Armstrong, spokesperson for the National Breast Implant Plaintiffs' Coalition, Dallas, Texas, to the MDL Plaintiffs' Steering Committee and the MDL Defendants' Legal Counsel Committee.

16. Thomas M. Burton, "Breast implant firms to settle for $4 billion," *The Wall Street Journal,* 14 February 1994, sec. A, p. 3.

17. Gina Kolata, "3 Companies in Landmark Accord on Lawsuits over breast implants," *New York Times,* 24 March 1994, sec. A, p. 1.

18. Los Angeles Times Service, "Breast-implant settlement clears major hurdle," *The Miami Herald,* 5 April 1994, sec. A, p. 4. See also (*The Washington Post*), "Implant settlement passes court hurdle," The Ft. Lauderdale *Sun Sentinel,* 5 April, 1993, sec. A, p. 4.

# GLOSSARY

adenocarcinoma: a malignant glandular cancer.

adrenal gland: a tiny gland located above each of the kidneys that produces import hormones such as cortisone, adrenalin, and aldosterone.

adjuvant: a nonspecific stimulator of the immune system.

amyotrophic lateral sclerosis (Lou Gehrig disease): a disease, usually fatal within two to three years, which is marked by progressive degeneration of brain and spinal neurons resulting in the wasting of muscles.

anesthesia: a loss of feeling, as in drug-induced to permit the performance of surgery.

angiosarcoma (hemangiosarcoma): a malignant tumor formed by proliferation of endothelial fibroblastic cells.

antibody: a circulating immunoglobulin, which is a protein molecule in the blood that interacts with an antigen.

antigen: any substance, which the host recognizes as a foreign (not itself), capable of inducing a specific immune response, as well as reacting with the product of that response, which is the antibody, lymphocyte, or both.

antigenic response: an immune response to an antigen.

antinuclear antibody (ANA): an antibody destructive to or reactive with components of the cell nucleus.

antiseptic: a substance that prevents decay.

aorta: the main vascular trunk leading from the heart from which the arterial (blood) system proceeds.

arthralgia: a pain in a joint.

arthritis: an inflammation of the connective-tissue structure of the joints.

asbestos: a fibrous, incombustible magnesium and calcium silicate used as thermal insulation, which can cause cancer.

asymptomatic: showing or causing no symptoms.

atrophy: a wasting away; a diminution of the size of a cell, tissue, organ, or part.

augmentation mammaplasty: a surgical procedure which increases the size and volume of a breast with the insertion of an implant (prosthesis) into the breast.

autoantibody: an abnormal antibody directed against a component of the same organism.

autoimmune disease: a disease caused by the immune response to the body's own tissue constituents (self antigens or autoantigens).

auxiliary: affording aid; that which affords aid.


bacteria: in general, unicellular microorganisms that commonly multiply by cell division (fission), some are capable of causing human illness.

benign: non-cancerous.

biochemical: pertaining to the chemistry of living organisms and of vital processes.

"bleed": leakage and escape of silicone gel through the porous, outer-envelope shell of a silicone gel-filled breast implant.

capsular contracture: the formation of a constricting fibrous layer, a scar capsule, around a breast implant as a result of an immune reaction to the foreign body (silicone) by the host.

carcinogen: any cancer-producing substance.

catalyst: a substance used to activate and achieve a desired chemical reaction.

Cat scan (computed axial tomography): a recording of internal body images by registering electronic impulses on a magnetic disk which is then processed and reconstructed for display by a mini-computer.

Cellular immunity: immunity mediated by T-lymphocytes either through the release of lymphokines or through exertion of direct cytotoxicity; transmissible by the transfer of lymphocytes but not serum. It comprises delayed hypersensitivity reactions, systemic response to viral and microbial infections, contact dermatitis, granulomatous reactions, graft versus host reactions, and other reactions.

chromosome: a structure in the nucleus of a cell containing a thread of DNA that transmits genetic information.

closed capsulotomy: a non-surgical procedure performed to break up the contracted scar capsule surrounding an implant by the application of external compression, a forceful squeezing of the breast.

collagen: the protein substance of the white fibers (collagenous fibers) of the skin, tendons, bone, cartilage, and all other connective tissue; composed of molecules of tropocollagen, which is the molecular unit of collagen fibrils, rich in glycine, proline, hydroproline, and hydroxylysine.

concomitant: accompanying; joined by another.

connective-tissue disease: a group of clinically distinct diseases that have in common widespread pathologic changes in the connective tissues of the body (bone, joint, muscle, tendon, ligament, skin, and covering tissues).

constitutional: affecting the make-up or functional habit of the body as a whole; not local.

cyclic: the term is applied to chemical compounds containing a ring of atoms in the nucleus; (closed chain), atoms linked together forming a ring that may be saturated or unsaturated (aromatic).

cytotoxic: having the ability to destroy cells.

defendant: the person or entity accused and sued in a legal action.

dermatomyositis: polymyositis occurring in association with characteristic inflammatory skin changes, including violaceous (violet-colored) papules over the knuckles; a violaceous or heliotrope (violet-colored) rash on the upper eyelids accompanied by edema; and an erythematous rash on the forehead, neck, shoulders, trunk, and arms.

DES: diethylstilbestrol, synthetic estrogen.

dioxin: any of the heterocyclic hydrocarbons presented as a trace contaminant in herbicides, especially the chlorinated dioxin 2, 3, 7, 8 tetrachlorodibenzo-para-dioxin, which is thought to have oncogenic and teratogenic properties.

DNA: a nucleic acid that constitutes the genetic material of the cellular organism.

dose-response: a reaction achieved by and relevant to the amount of a chemical, drug administered in treatment.

edema: the presence of abnormally large amounts of fluid in the intercellular tissue spaces of the body.

EEG (electroencephalogram): a recording of brain waves generating from currents emanating from nerve cells in the brain.

embryo: the product of the developing, fertilized ovum, beginning about two weeks after fertilization to the end of the seventh or eighth week, which will eventually become the fetus.

encephalopathy: an unspecified brain disorder.

endocarditis: an inflammation of the endocardium, a membrane lining the cavities of the heart and connective-tissue bed on which it lies.

endocrine: applied to organs and structures whose function is to secrete into the blood or lymph a substance (hormone) that has specific function on another organ or part.

endocrinologic: pertaining to the endocrine system.

endometriosis: a condition in which tissue resembling the uterine mucous membrane occurs abnormally in various locations in the pelvic cavity.

erythematous: characterized by erythema, which is a name applied to redness of the skin produced by a congestion of the capillaries (minute blood vessels) resulting from a variety of causes.

estrogen: female sex hormones produced by the ovaries (may possibly be produced by the adrenals, placenta, and fat).

enzyme: a protein molecule that catalyzes chemical reactions of other substances without itself being destroyed or altered upon completion of the reactions.


febrile: pertaining to or characterized by fever.

fetotoxic: a substance poisonous to a developing fetus.

fetus: the unborn offspring in the post-embryonic period, seven to eight weeks after fertilization, until birth.

fibromyalgia: a condition consisting of diffuse muscle pain and weakness, which is not attributable to other known causes.

fibrosarcoma: an extremely lethal soft-tissue malignancy derived from the fibroblast, connective tissue cells, which produce collagen.

fibrotic: pertaining to or characterized by fibrosis, the formation or degeneration of fibrous tissue.

fibrous: composed of or containing fibers.

foreign body reaction: an immune response to a foreign substance, one not recognized by the body as "self."

fungus(i): a general term used to denote a group of eukaryotic protists, a single cell organism with a true nucleus, including mushrooms, yeasts, rusts, molds, etc.


Gallium scan: (nuclear medicine) a scan requiring an injection of a radioisotope, gallium, to image the soft tissue of the body, such as the lungs and the lymph nodes.

gamma globulin: a fraction of the serum containing immunoglobulins, which are proteins that may function as antibodies.

gangrene: the death of tissue, usually in considerable mass and associated with the loss of vascular supply, followed by bacterial invasion.

gene: a segment of a DNA molecule that contains all of the information required for the synthesis of a product, including both coding and non-coding sequences.

glomerular lesions: a lesion, which is a pathological tissue abnormality, or loss of function of a part, involving part of the kidney.

glycoprotein: a conjugated class of proteins, consisting of a compound of protein with a carbohydrate group.

granuloma: a non-cancerous lump or nodule consisting of inflammatory cells or a collection of modified macrophages representing a chronic, inflammatory response initiated by various agents.


hapten: a small molecule, not antigenic by itself, that can react with antibodies of appropriate specificity and elicit the formation of such antibodies when conjugated to a larger antigenic molecule, usually a protein, called in this context the carrier.

Hashimoto's thyroiditis: a progressive autoimmune disease of the thyroid.

hemodialysis: the removal of certain elements from the blood by virtue of the difference in the rates of their diffusion through a semipermeable membrane by means of a machine (hemodialyzer).

hepatic: pertaining to the liver.

hormones: a chemical substance, produced in the body by an organ, or cells of an organ, which as a specific regulatory effect on the activity of a certain organ or organs; originally applied to substances secreted by various endocrine glands and transported in the blood system to the distant target organ on which their effect was produced. The term was later applied to various substances not produced by special glands but having similar action, both locally and anatomically remote.

humoral immunity: immunity that is mediated by antibodies through the blood.

hypercalcemia: an excess of calcium in the blood.

hyperplasia: the abnormal multiplication or increase in the number of normal cells in the normal arrangement of tissue.

hyperplastic: representing hyperplasia.

hypersensitivity: a state of altered reactivity in which the body reacts with an exaggerated immune response.

hypervolemia: an abnormal increase in the volume of circulating fluid (plasma) in the blood.

hysterectomy: the surgical removal of the uterus.

immune response: the body's response to a foreign invader in an attempt to provide immunity, protection against disease.

immunoglobulin: any of the structurally-related serum proteins that function as antibodies.

infection: the invasion and multiplication of microorganisms in the body tissue.

inflammation: a localized, protective response elicited by injury or destruction of tissues, which serves to destroy, dilute, or wall off both the injurious agent and the injured tissue.

interoperative: occurring during the course of a surgical operation.

intramuscular: within the substance of a muscle.

interuterine: within the uterus.

invasive cancers: ones that have the ability to spread from the site of origin to adjoining tissues.

intubation: the insertion of a tube into a body canal or hollow organ.

in utero: within the uterus.

isotope: a chemical element having the same atomic number as another but possessing a different mass.

lactation: the secretion of milk.

latency: a period during which a disease is dormant after exposure to an infectious or toxic substance before initiating signs of active disease.

lesion: any pathological or traumatic discontinuity of tissue or loss of function of a part.

Leukemia: a progressive, malignant disease of the white-cell blood-forming organs.

leukocyte: a white blood cell or corpuscle.

lipid: any of a group of fat or fat-like substances that are easily stored by the body and which are important constituents of cell structure. Lipids include fatty acids, neutral fats, waxes, and steroids.

litigant: any party involved in a lawsuit.

lupus erythematosus, systemic: a chronic, remitting, and relapsing inflammation and often febrile, multisystemic disorder of the connective tissue which may be acute or insidious in onset, characterized primarily by involvement of the skin, joints, kidneys, and serosal membranes.

lymphadenitis: an inflammation of one or more lymph nodes, usually caused by a primary focus of infection elsewhere.

lymphadenoma: lymphoma, which is the abnormal cell multiplication of lymphoid tissue or lymphatic cancer that may be malignant.

lymphadenopathy: enlarged and/or diseased lymph nodes.

lymphatic system: the vessels which collect lymph, a transparent, yellowish liquid derived from all tissue fluids from all parts of the body, and then return it to the blood.

lymph node: a filtering gland made up of lymphatic tissue which are located throughout the body and which aid in defending against foreign invaders by inhibiting their entrance into the bloodstream.

lymphocyte: a mononuclear, nonphagocytic leukocyte found in the blood, lymph, and lymphoid tissue that is responsible for humoral and cellular immunity.

lymphokine: a general term for soluble mediators of immune responses that are not antibodies or complement components and are released by sensitized lymphocytes upon contact with an antigen.

Lymphoma: malignant cancer of the lymphatic system.

macrophages: phagocytic white cells which act as part of the immune response and engulf foreign invaders.

malignant: tending to become progressively worse and to result in death; cancerous, having properties of invasion and metastasis.

mammogram: a radiograph of the breast.

mammaplasty: plastic surgical reconstruction of a breast to augment or reduce its size.

mastectomy: the surgical removal of a breast.

mastopathy: disease of the mammary gland.

mediated: indirect, accomplished by the aid of an intervening medium.

menopausal: pertaining to the cessation of menstruation.

Mesothelioma: a malignant connective-tissue sarcoma.

metabolism: the sum of all the physical and chemical processes by which living organized substance is produced and maintained; also the transformation by which energy is made available for the uses of the organism.

metastasis: the spread of cancer cells to other organs not directly connected to the cancerous organ via the blood system.

microadenoma: an adenoma, a benign tumor in which the cells form recognizable glandular structures, as of the anterior pituitary, less than 10 mm in diameter.

microorganism: a very tiny, microscopic, individual, living thing, whether a plant or an animal.

morbidity: a diseased condition or state.

MRI: magnetic resonance imaging.

multi-focal: a process of disease involving many areas.

multiple sclerosis: a usually prolonged, relapsing disease in which there are patches of demyelination (the destruction or loss of myelin) throughout the white matter of the central nervous system, which sometimes extends into the gray matter.

mutagenic: a substance that induces genetic mutation (changes).

myalgia: pain in the muscle.

myelopathy: functional disturbances and/or pathological changes in the spinal cord.

myelin: a substance with a high proportion of lipid to protein that forms a protective sheath surrounding the nerves.

myositis: an inflammatory, progressive disease of a voluntary muscle.

necrosis: the death of cells caused by the progressive degradation actions of enzymes.

neoplasm: any new and abnormal growth, specifically a new growth of tissue in which the growth is uncontrolled and progressive.

neuralgia: pain that extends along the course of one or more nerves.

neuropathy: a general term denoting functional disturbances and/or pathological changes in the peripheral nervous system.

neurotoxicity: the quality of exerting a poisonous effect upon the nerve issue.

oncogenes: a gene found in the chromosomes of tumor cells whose activation is associated with the initial and continuing conversion of normal cells into cancer cells.

ovariectomy: (oophorectomy) the surgical removal of the ovaries.

ovary: one of two female sexual glands in which the ova (eggs) are formed.

ovulation: the discharge of a secondary oocyte (a developing egg of two states) from the ovary.

ovum: the femal reproductive cell (egg).

oxidation: a chemical process consisting of the increase of positive charges on an atom or the loss of negative charges.

paresthesia: an abnormal sensation (such as burning or prickling).

parotid: a salivary gland situated between the ear and chin.

pathology: the structural and functional manifestations of disease.

peripheral: pertaining to the outward part, surface, or structure; situated away rom a center or central structure.

peritoneal cavity: the abdominal cavity.

peritoneum: the serous membrane lining the abdominal-pelvic walls and the abdominal cavity.

peroxidase: an enzyme that catalyzes the oxidation of a substance with a reduction of hydrogen peroxide.

placenta: an organ joining mother and child, which provides nourishment to the embryo/fetus.

phagocytosis: the process by which macrophages engulf foreign invaders.

pituitary gland: a small gland consisting of two lobes, located at the base of the brain and attached by a stack to the hypothalamus; this unit is of vital importance to growth, maturation, and reproduction of the individual.

plaintiff: one who files a lawsuit against another person or entity.

PMA: pre-market approval, one of three classifications of medical devices requiring the submission of safety date to the FDA in order to market a product.

polyarthralgia: pain involving many joints.

polymyositis: a chronic, progressive inflammatory disease of skeletal muscles characterized by symmetrical weakness of the limb girdles (encircling structures), neck, and pharynx, usually associated with pain and tenderness.

progesterone: a female hormone, part of the normal process of uterine physiology, which is produced in the ovary, as well as adrenal glands and placenta, whose function is to prepare the uterus for the reception and development of the fertilized ovum.

prognosis: a prediction concerning, especially, the course of a disease.

prosthesis: an artificial substitute for a missing part of the body, either for functional or cosmetic purposes.

protocol: an explicit, detailed plan of an experiment.

protoplasm: the essential material of all plant and animal cells consisting of nucleic acids, proteins, lipids, carbohydrates, and inorganic salts.

pulmonary: pertaining to the lungs.

purpura: a small hemorrhage in the skin, mucous membranes, or serosal surface that may be caused by various factors including blood disorders, vascular abnormalities, and trauma.

radioisotope scanning: the production of a two-dimensional picture representing the gamma rays emitted by a radioactive isotope concentration in specific tissue in the body.

Raynaud's syndrome: an idiopathic hypersensitivity to cold which is a vascular disorder characterized by a constriction of the blood vessels in the fingers and toes, sometimes the ears and nose, and often accompanied by pain; the disorder causes intermittent attacks of pallor followed by cyanosis (a darkening, a duskiness), then redness of the affected areas. The attacks are initiated by exposure to cold or emotional disturbance.

rheumatic: pertaining to or affected by rheumatism, which is a disease marked by inflammation and degeneration or metabolic derangement of connective-tissue structures of the body, especially the joints and their related structures.

rheumatoid arthritis: a chronic, inflammatory, and systemic disease primarily of the joints, which may result in deformity and immobility of the affected joints.


salivary: pertaining to the glands (the parotid, submaxillary, sublingual, and smaller mucous glands of the mouth), which excrete saliva, a clean, alkaline secretion which softens and moistens foods and contains amylase, a digestive enzyme.

sarcoid: a tumor, often highly malignant, made up of a substance like the embryonic connective tissue; which is composed of closely packed cells embedded in a homogeneous (consisting of similar elements) substance.

Scheie Syndrome: the mildest of three allelic (alternative gene) disorders resulting in the defective degradation of mucopolysaccharide sulfates, which then accumulate in the tissue; the disorder is characterized by corneal clouding, claw hand, and the involvement of the aortic valve.

scleroderma: the chronic hardening and thickening of the skin, which may be found in several different diseases and occurs in either localized or systemic form.

sclerosis: an induration or hardening of a part caused by inflammation and, in diseases of the nervous system, due to hyperplasia of the connective tissue or to designate hardening of the blood vessels.

serous: pertaining to or resembling serum.

silica: silicone dioxide, $SiO_2$, or silicic anhydride, occurring in nature as agate, amethyst, sand, quartz, chalcedony, cristobalite, and flint.

silicate: a salt of any of the silicic acids, which occur in hydrated forms of silica.

silicon: a nonmetallic element occurring in nature as silica.

silicone: any organic compound in which all or part of the carbon has been replaced with silicon.

silicosis: a progressive and usually fatal disease caused by pneumoconiosis (the permanent deposition of substantial particulate matter in the lungs) due to the breathing of silica dust, which results in the formation of generalized nodular fibrotic changes in both lungs.

Sjogren's Syndrome: a disease marked by a lacrimal (tear) deficiency with or without lacrimal and salivary gland enlargement and the presence of connective-tissue disease.

sonogram: the visualization of deep structures of the body by recording the reflections of pulses of ultrasonic waves directed into the body.

SPEC (Single Proton Computed Tomography): a nuclear medicine scan that requires a radioisotope injection; frequently used to image the bone, heart, and brain.

sphincteric: pertaining to or resembling a ringlike band of fibers that constrict a passage or close off a natural orifice.

spleen: a large, glandlike but ductless organ situated in the upper-left abdominal cavity; the largest structure of the lymphoid (lymph) system.

splenic: pertaining to the spleen.

subcutaneous: beneath the skin.

synovitis: an inflammation of the synovial membrane, a protective sheath covering the tendons.

systemic: pertaining to or affecting the body as a whole.

systemic scleroderma: (systemic sclerosis) a systemic disorder of the connective tissue characterized by induration and thickening of the skin by abnormalities of both the smaller and larger blood vessels, and by fibrotic degenerative changes in various body organs.

teratogen: an agent or factor that causes the production of physical defects in the developing embryo/fetus.

toxicology: the scientific study of poison, their actions, their detection, and the treatment of conditions caused by them.

trauma: a wound or injury.

tumor: a swelling; one of the cardinal signs of inflammation; a diseased enlargement.

tumorigenesis: the production of tumors.

ultrasonography: the visualization of deep structures within the body by recording the reflections (echoes) of pulses of ultrasonic waves.

<u>ureter</u>: the fibromuscular tube that conveys the urine from the kidney to the bladder.

<u>uterine</u>: pertaining to the uterus.

<u>uterus</u>: a hollow muscular organ in female mammals in which the fertilized ovum becomes embedded and in which the developing embryo and fetus are nourished.

<u>vacuole</u>: any space or cavity within the protoplasm of a cell.

<u>vascular</u>: pertaining to the blood vessels.

# BIBLIOGRAPHY

## I. Books

Brunning, Nancy. *Breast Implants: Everything You Want To Know.* Alameda, CA: Hunter House, Inc., Publishers, 1992.

Lappé, Marc. *Chemical Deceptions.* San Francisco, CA: Sierra Club Books, 1991.

Love, Susan M. *Dr. Susan Love's Breast Book.* Reading, MA: Addison-Wesley Publishing Company, 1990.

Rubin, Leonard R., editor. *Biomaterials in Reconstructive Surgery.* St. Louis, MO: The C.V. Mosby Company, 1983.

Samter, Max, editor. *Immunological Diseases.* Boston, MA: Little, Brown and Company, 1988.

Sacarello, Hildegarde L.A. *The Comprehensive Handbook of Hazardous Materials.* Boca Raton, FL: Lewis Publishers, 1993.

Vasey, Frank B. and Feldstein, Josh. *The Silicone Implant Controversy.* Freedom, CA: The Crossing Press, 1993.

Wolfe, Sidney. *Woman's Health Alert.* Reading, MA: Addison-Wesley Publishing Company, 1991.

# TORN ILLUSIONS

## II. Articles and Reports

Berkman, Leslie. "The Silicone Controversy." *Los Angeles Times*, December 1990.

Boca Raton Hotel and Health Club. "Report on the ATLA Convention Breast Implant Litigation Group Seminar." Boca Raton, FL. 22 January 1992

Castleman, Michael. "Women's Warrior." *California Lawyer*, March 1993, pp. 45-106.

Datan, Nancy. "Illness and Imagery: Female Cognition, Socialization, and Gender Identity." *Gender and Thought: Psychological Prospectives*, New York: Stringer-Verlay, 1989.

Davis, Lisa. "The Implant Panic." *Vogue*, May 1992, pp. 166-170.

David, Lisa. "Vanities." *Health*, September/October 1991, pp. 30-34.

Drawbridge, Jennifer. "Implants: Dangerous Curves." *Mirabella*, August 1992, pp. 52-58.

Duckman, Linda. "A Healing Choice." *Self*, January 1990.

Francis, Pam. "Turning Toxic Breasts into Gold." *The Houston Press*, January 1993, pp. 14-21

Fraser, Laura. "The Cosmetic Surgery Hoax." *Glamour*, February 1990, pp. 184-233.

"Global Settlement Negotiations conducted in Secret." *Mealey's Litigation Report*, 8 April 1993.

Goldrich, Sybil Niden. "Restoration." *MS*, June 1988.

Human Resources and Intergovernmental Relations Subcommittee of the Committee on Government Operations (The). "The FDA's Regulation of Silicone Breast Implants." Washington: U.S. Government Printing Office, 1993.

Jones, Abbie. "Implant Impact: European Health Officials Question FDA Ban." *Today's Boca Women*, September 1992, pp. 17-19.

Jones, Jane S. "The Dangers of Breast Augmentation." *The Network News*, July/August 1989.

Long, Karen R. "Breast-Implant Industry Stung By Safety Fears." *Health and Science*, 11 June 1991.

"Multidistrict Litigation Ordered for Breast Implant Cases." *The ATLA Advocate*, 18 (7) August 1992.

National Women's Health Resource Center. *Breast Implants Special Report*, 14 (2) March/April 1992, pp.1-9.

Peters, Douglas and Aulion, Margaret M. "Breast Implants: Science and Litigation." *Trial*, November 1991, pp. 26-32.

Podolsky, Doug. "Breast Implants: What Price Vanity?" *American Health*, March 1991, pp. 70-75.

Purvis, Andrew. "Time Bombs in the Breasts." *Time,* April 1991, p. 70.

Regush, Nicholas. "Toxic Breasts." *Mother Jones,* January/February 1992, pp. 25-31.

Rohlfing, Carla. "Is There a Time Bomb Ticking in Women's Chests?" *Longevity,* July 1991, pp. 52-58.

Rome, Ester R. "Are Breast Implants Really Safe?" *Sojourner: The Women's Forum,* November 1989.

Rome, Ester R. "Silicone Breast Implants." *Middlesex News,* 1990.

Rome, Ester R. "Unconventional Wisdom." *The Women's Review of Books,* 8 (4) January 1991.

Salmans, Sandra. "Women's Health Alert: How Safe Are Breast Implants? Here Are the Facts Every Woman Should Know." *Ladies Home Journal,* July 1991, p. 44.

Seligmen, Jean with Church, Vernon. "A Vote of No Confidence." *Newsweek,* March 1992: p.75

Smart, Tim. "Breast Implants: What Did the Industry Know, and When?" *Business Week,* June 1991, pp. 94-98.

United District Court, Northern District Alabama, Southern Division, before Honorable Sam C. Pointer, Jr. "Transcript: Silicone Gel Breast Implants Hearing (no. CV 92-P-10000-S). Products Liability Litigation (MDL-926)." 24 February 1993.

United States Food and Drug Administration - various memorandums, *Federal register* publications, notices, panel reviews, transcripts, and circulations.

Vallbona, Nuri. "What Price Beauty?" *The Houston Post,* 7 July 1991.

Wilkenson, Paula. "General Silicone Chemistry." *Chemical Engineer,* Breast Implant Task Force, U.S. Food and Drug Administration. Undated (Obtained February 1992).

### III. Information Packets and Newsletters

BIFF, Breast Implant Information Center
Boston Women's Health Book Collective
Coalition of Silicone Survivors
Command Trust Network
National Women's Health Network
National Women's Health Resource Center
Public Citizens Health Research Group
TBIF, Breast Implant Information Foundation